Maria Tita Portal Sacramento
Marcelo Williams Oliveira de Souza

Nursing in health: Experiences of undergraduate students

Maria Tita Portal Sacramento
Marcelo Williams Oliveira de Souza

Nursing in health: Experiences of undergraduate students

In the state of Pará

ScienciaScripts

Imprint

Cover image: www.ingimage.com

This book is a translation from the original published under ISBN 978-3-330-75673-1.

Publisher:
Sciencia Scripts
is a trademark of
Dodo Books Indian Ocean Ltd. and OmniScriptum S.R.L publishing group

120 High Road, East Finchley, London, N2 9ED, United Kingdom
Str. Armeneasca 28/1, office 1, Chisinau MD-2012, Republic of Moldova, Europe
Printed at: see last page
ISBN: 978-620-8-28070-3

CONTENTS

ORGANIZERS

MARIA TITA PORTAL SACRAMENTO

> PhD in Nursing. Anna Nery Nursing School, EEAN, Brazil.

> Master in Nursing. Paulista School of Medicine, EPM, Brazil.

> Specialist in Pedagogical Training in Professional Education. Faculty of Nursing, University of Rio de Janeiro, UERJ, Brazil.

> Specialist in Occupational Nursing. Magalhaes Barata Nursing School, EEMB/FUNDACENTRO, Brazil.

> Specialist in Obstetric Nursing. Paulista School of Medicine/UNIFESP, Brazil.

> Training in Public Health. University of Sao Paulo, USP, Brazil. Degree in Nursing. Magalhaes Barata Nursing School, EMB/UEPA, Brazil.

> Degree in Nursing from the Magalhaes Barata School of Nursing/EEMB-UEPA.

> Retired lecturer at the State University of Parà. Magalhaes Barata Nursing School (1966 - 2000).

> Nursing Assistant at the Ministry of Health (1966 - 2000).

> Coordinator of the Nursing Course at the University of Amazonia/UNAMA (2008 - 2015).

> Current coordinator of the Nursing Degree Course at Faculdade da Amazônia/FAAM.

MARCELO WILLIAMS OLIVEIRA DE SOUZA

> Master's student in the National Network in Environmental Science Teaching. Federal University of Parà, UFPA, Brazil.

> Specializing in Quality and Patient Safety. Sirio Libanês Institute, ISL, Brazil.

> Specialist in Nephrology and Urology Nursing. Higher School of Amazonia, ESAMAZ, Brazil.

> Specialist in Intensive Care Nursing: Adult and Neonatal. Metropolitan College of Amazonia - FAMAZ, Brazil.

> Further training in Youth, Sexuality and STD/AIDS Prevention. Federal University of Parà, UFPA, Brazil.

> Training in Pedagogical Competence for the Practice of Preceptorship. Brazilian

Association of Medical Education, ABEM, Brazil.

> Degree in Nursing. University of Amazonia, UNAMA, Brazil.

> Preceptor for the Nursing Degree Course at the University of Amazonia.

> Lecturer in the Postgraduate Course at the Escola Superior da Amazônia/ESAMAZ.

> Assistant Nurse at the Intensive Care Unit of the Santa Casa de Misericòrdia do Parà Foundation/FSCMP.

> He worked as an Assistance Nurse at the Metropolitan Urgency and Emergency Hospital and at the Unimed Belém General Hospital.

PRESENTATION

Nursing is a profession committed to the health of the human being and the community. It works to promote, protect, recover health and rehabilitate people, respecting ethical and legal precepts. The nursing professional participates as a member of society and in actions aimed at satisfying the health needs of the population, respecting the life, dignity and rights of the human person.

Nurses have three different roles in today's context: **actors in training and trainers:** as actors in training they must be constantly learning to meet the needs of society and as trainers they are responsible for training future professionals, as well as health education, as a bridge to promoting the health of each client. There is also a commitment to research. **Political Actor**: Nurses are not very active, so they need to become aware of their role as active subjects in relationships and start acting in the political field, by participating in the formulation of health policies and in the management of the health system. **Actor of Care**: The nurse is now one of the main protagonists of the health system, and is responsible for assisting clients, monitoring progress and desired results, developing the interdisciplinary care plan and improving quality and safety, covering primary care, long-term care, home care and palliative care.

We emphasize the importance of the nursing professional within the context of health, based on the principle that caring for human beings necessarily requires looking at the total dimension of the being, including its existential essence. According to the Brazilian Dr. Wanda Horta, nursing is "the science and art of assisting human beings (individuals, families and communities) in meeting their basic needs". In other words, nurses are taking on an increasingly decisive and proactive role in identifying the care needs of the population, as well as in promoting and protecting the health of individuals in their different dimensions.

In public health, nurses are the coordinators of most of the Ministry of Health's programs. In this area of health promotion and prevention, nurses are responsible for educating people to change their individual and community lifestyles in order to improve their quality of life.

Given this comprehensive importance, I see nursing as the guiding force behind a consistent and organized care process. I also see nursing as the protagonist of the health system, and so I realize the need to study it more and more in a targeted way.

You have to study in the knowledge that your technical and scientific knowledge can change the health history of Brazil, especially that of each of our patients. Studying contributes to the development of our profession and is the only way to become a valued professional. In this book we will focus on nursing care, with research carried out in this area of knowledge.

The nursing staff are the ones who spend the most time with the patient and their family, they are the ones who provide the most care and, consequently, they are also the ones who keep the most records in the patient's chart.

Nursing notes are used both to obtain information about the care given to patients, guaranteeing quality and safety in the continuity of nursing care and that of the multidisciplinary team, and for the legal support/protection of professionals. The lack of these records or inadequate records can compromise patient care and cause great harm to the nursing team and the institution.

When we talk about nursing notes, we inevitably think about how important they are for supporting the nurse in the care plan, as they are one of the instruments we use to evaluate the results of the care prescribed and already given, to assess the patient's progress and the need to maintain or change strategies in order to achieve the established goals. In view of this, we can say that good nursing notes help us to develop an excellent Systematization of Nursing Care (SNC).

The inclusion of fathers in prenatal care is a reproductive right. In addition to being one of the most important moments for establishing an early bond between father and child, it is also considered a way of preventing domestic violence against children and family abandonment.

The importance of a father's presence at prenatal consultations is essential, as he can provide support for the woman, creating security and tranquillity during the pregnancy and also increasing his knowledge of how to care for the woman's health and that of her future child. Paternity gives men recognition of their masculinity, and by taking on paternity they also acquire responsibility and assume the consequences of their attitudes.

Fatherhood should not only be seen from a legal reproductive point of view, but above all as a man's right to participate in the whole process, from the decision of whether or not to have children, to how and when to have them, as well as monitoring pregnancy, childbirth, the postpartum period and the child's upbringing. The experience of fatherhood also depends on the relationship lived between father and child in the past, which influences the way men understand and assume their masculinity in order to fulfill themselves as fathers.

Among the main problems related to the use of medicines in hospital units are drug interactions (DI), which, when not prevented or treated promptly, can cause irreparable damage to the patient. Studies show that DIs are frequent in ICU patients, with higher rates than in patients hospitalized in other units'

From a professional point of view, the nursing team has a unique role to play in preventing MIs, as it is responsible for scheduling, preparing, administering and monitoring the effects of medicines. However, it is essential that they are aware of and know how to identify possible MIs so as not to expose patients to unwanted situations.

Finally, considering that knowledge of drug interactions is an important tool for optimizing nursing care, this study was carried out with the aim of analyzing nurses' knowledge of drug interactions.

Different perspectives on humanization are already known and applied, but humanizing the nursing profession is in line with the ethical and legal precepts that govern the profession. Because the environment of the Neonatal Intensive Care Unit (NICU) generates various feelings of fear, insecurity and ambivalence in both parents and professionals, it is essential to humanize the workers who work in the sector, respecting their ethical position in order to achieve better results.

The presence of humanized care in this environment becomes relevant, being perceived as working in harmony between the various technologies; technical and scientific knowledge, with respect and appreciation of the human being and their differences and singularities in an integral way.

Humanized care must be given in such a way as to attribute citizenship and solidarity to the diversity of each individual, emphasizing their subjectivity and satisfying their needs and those of the professionals who assist the users of these services.

The search by professionals for an affective interpersonal relationship, in the sense of interaction between the team itself, the family and the patient, is significant for the humanization of the care provided. Communication is the main means of interaction, listening, commitment to the emotional state and respect for the patient's autonomy help to respond to their wishes.

This is why we decided to write this book, considering that there are several factors that may at first appear as weaknesses and that may influence the applicability of scientific, technological and humanized nursing care. In addition, the professional's own perception of the subject could help the nursing team to provide qualified nursing care.

MARIA TITA PORTAL SACRAMENTO MARCELO WILLIAMS OLIVEIRA DE SOUZA

CHAPTER I - THE IMPORTANCE OF RECORDS FOR NURSING: ANOTATION AND EVOLUTION

ABEL DOS SANTOS

LARISSA NASCIMENTO AZEVEDO DA SILVA

MARCELO DOS SANTOS MIRANDA

MARIA TITA PORTAL SACRAMENTO

SUMMARY

Nursing note-taking is a multidisciplinary practice that requires constant updating and a lot of attention when transcribing to the medical record, because the records describe everything that happens in the process of patient development, be it of a clinical, administrative or legal ethical nature. In healthcare institutions, the nursing team is responsible for this process, supported by the Professional Practice Law No. 7.498/96, but in Brazil there is a lack of value placed on nursing notes. With this in mind, we sought to analyze the nursing notes and evolutions in the medical clinic sector of a private hospital in Belèm do Parâ. The research had a qualitative and exploratory descriptive approach. Data was collected from the medical records of 10 patients admitted to the medical clinic over a period of one week to one month, during the months of August and September, and analyzed using the content analysis method. The profile of the patients in the medical records analyzed showed that they ranged in age from 30 to 94, and that the majority were male. We observed that 80% of the notes were legible, clear and objective; all the records did not contain any of the following items: date, time, signature or identification of the professional, the lack of date and time being the most recurrent factors, in 90% of cases there were erasures, blank lines and spaces; and 80% contained only abbreviations provided for in the literature, 90% contained the care provided and records of the advice and information given; however, 100% did not present the patient's response to this care or descriptions of characteristics such as: measured size, quantity, color and shape, 90% did not contain terms that gave a connotation of value and 60% of the notes referred to simple data without further scientific study. It is considered that nursing notes are important for monitoring patients and observing the evolution of their clinical condition. The study shows that there is no concern on the part of nurses to keep records in accordance with the recommendations for auditing medical records.

Key words: Nursing records. Nursing notes.

Prompts.

1 INTRODUCTION

Nursing records explain all the existing data on the progress of patients, whether for clinical evaluation of the human being, or for legal administrative or ethical issues, they need scientific content, consistency and often meaning, because sometimes the notes are undervalued.

The nursing team is responsible for all the care to be carried out, observing basic ethical and moral principles, with a view to patient safety and privacy. The description of the care that will be carried out must be systematic, obeying all the criteria and standards established by COREN/SP (2011) for good care; systematically observing and evaluating the client in terms of possible variables in their behavior, as well as the possibility of care that is not being provided for a good progression in treatment. In this way, nursing plays an important role when it comes to making observations, as good progress will be of great importance in achieving therapeutic goals (HORTA, 1970).

Lack of nursing records can lead to losses for the hospital when it comes to charging its fees, as well as ineffective treatment due to a lack of follow-up by nursing staff, which tends to increase the length of hospitalization, increase the cost of treatment and cause greater morbidity for the patient (OGUISSO, 1975).

Nursing notes are one of the most important communication tools. This communication, whether through oral or written language, is essential for nursing practice (MATOS, 1997). Therefore, records are essential elements in the process of human care, and when they are written in a way that portrays the reality to be documented, they enable continuous communication and can be used for various purposes, such as: teaching; research; audits; legal proceedings; planning and others of interest related to this subject (MATSUDA, 2006).

The need for adequate and frequent records in the patient's chart is paramount. The notes recorded by the nursing team are the most important instrument for evaluating the quality of nursing care, and represent half of the information inherent in patient care recorded in the medical record (SANTOS, 2003).

Along the same lines, many authors have argued that nursing professionals do not give due importance to records as a source of communication, as a means of evaluating the care provided to patients and as a document that serves as proof of the application of nursing theories to practice (MATOS, 1997; SANTOS, 2003).

According to COREN/SP (2011) nursing notes are a professional practice (nurses, nursing technicians and nursing assistants). This process should require a great deal of responsibility and honesty when describing procedures and any other care carried out to provide comfort and well-being for the patient, as these descriptions will be of great importance for the cure or palliative treatment of their pathology.

Nurses are responsible for the early detection of possible risks and complications of treatment, in order to guarantee the patient's safety and well-being through the information recorded in the medical record. This is why laws have been established, and it is through these laws that the criteria for good nursing notes will be enforced, which must be clear, objective, precise, in legible handwriting, without erasures; chronological and written in ink (ballpoint pen), never in pencil (COREN/SP, 2011).

The nurse must know the patient in order to carry out possible nursing interventions. To do this, the nurse must be informed of their pathology and how their treatment is progressing, which will be based on what has been described in the medical record, in order to take measures that can stabilize the needs presented by the patient, which is why it is important to write down everything that happens to the patient 24 hours a day. It is therefore essential for nurses to have a broad view of nursing notes and each of their processes, in order to avoid possible errors that could result in harm to the patient (LOURENÇO, 2000).

2 JUSTIFICATION

During our internships as students, we observed the great difficulty the nursing team has when it comes to recording the care given to patients, because, in the healthcare institutions we visited, we were able to observe that there is a great difference between the records kept by the nursing team and those found in the literature.

The nursing course offers the subject of records and notes in the course of the subjects, creating skills for development in practice.

In nursing systematization, recording the procedures carried out gives us the security of quality care, because the nursing diagnosis and care prescriptions are then made.

Therefore, this study makes us reflect on the importance of nursing records to improve the patient's state of health, and it is essential that nurses supervise and evaluate the records of care provided. Supported by COFEN resolution 311/2007, which approves the new reformulation of the code of ethics for nursing professionals, which states in Art. 68 the duty to "record in the medical record and other documents specific to nursing, information relating to the process of caring for the person", valuing the work of the nursing team (BRASIL, 2007)".

3 OBJECTIVES

3.1 GENERAL OBJECTIVE

Analyze nursing notes and progress in the care of hospitalized patients.

3.2 SPECIFIC OBJECTIVES

- Check the nursing notes and progress in the medical records;
- To identify the main difficulties in the daily lives of the nursing team in relation to the knowledge and practice of nursing notes and evolutions;
- Identify the profile of the patients.

4 THEORETICAL BASIS

4.1 HISTORY OF NURSING RECORDS

Nursing notes are an important means of communication for the team, because as well as indicating the actions taken, they enable continuity of care (VENTURINE, 2008). In the hospital environment, for example, it includes the recording of the patient's progress during hospitalization, a fact that covers various aspects (subjective: feelings and emotions expressed by the patient; and objective: clinical data on the patient) and provides ethical and legal support for the professional responsible for the care, since it offers information on the care provided by the nursing team and administrative data (D"INNOCENZO, 2006).

There is great interest in studying the importance of nursing records. Over the years, several studies have been carried out on this subject. According to Nóbrega (1980), in a study carried out on EEUSP's *PeriEnf* database, the oldest article was published in 1957 in Revista Paulista de Hospitais, by nurse Irmâ Maria Lasi, head of the first men's clinic at Santa Casa de Misericórdia de Sâo Paulo. The author gives a brief summary of the history of the medical record, then goes on to discuss its usefulness in a hospital environment and points out that among the many benefits of this type of documentation, the most important is its contribution to the progress of medical science and that a well-organized medical record makes it easier for the doctor to analyze and act with the patient (CARRIJO, 2006*)*.

In the 1970s, according to research carried out by Carrijo (2006), six more articles were published. These reaffirmed the importance of the nursing record, especially the notes, highlighting it as an instrument for evaluating the quality of care provided. In the 1980s, fourteen articles were published highlighting the issue of auditing and the content of nursing records, with a slight increase in the 1990s, when 16 articles were analyzed.

Finally, in the current decade of this millennium, we can see that there is greater and greater interest in these aspects, based on previous studies in various specific areas of nursing practice (CARRIJO, 2006). However, we found no studies relating to nursing records in clinical medicine.

Thus, the scarcity of studies related to nursing notes during the care of patients undergoing treatment in the medical clinic is a worldwide problem, which reinforces the importance of new studies that make it possible to reliably record information about the care provided to patients and how care is provided in the medical clinic.

42 THE NURSING NOTE

Nursing notes can be beneficial and fundamental in various pathologies, for example, in the treatment of severe hypertension, which requires strict control in order to reduce blood pressure more effectively, since the notes provided in the medical record will be indispensable for the treatment, which will provide a balance and stability for the patient's improvement (CIANCIARULLO, 1996).

The responses resulting from nursing notes can lead to a reduction in the effectiveness of the treatment, simply because of the lack of communication, thus jeopardizing the continuity of the treatment, leaving unfavorable responses not foreseen in the patient's improvement (wrong notes), which can cause numerous sequelae or even lead to death, depending on the degree of severity, or even cause no change in the desired care (DANIEL, 1983).

These notes also generate documents that allow members of the healthcare team to become aware of the decisions, actions and results obtained from the care provided; in addition to providing information, this documentation serves as a research tool and also as an ethical/legal instrument, making it possible to evaluate the quality of the care provided to the patient, as well as serving as a source of data for audits (DIAS, 1999).

In practice, the issue of note-taking is complex, because nurses, technicians and assistants end up confused about who is responsible for making the notes and how to do it, because the technicians make the notes and the nurses make the progress, which ends up generating confusing and unimportant information for the medical record, This often leads to a delay in improvement or even worsening due to the lack of communication between the teams, causing problems that could be avoided in order to provide good patient care (TONG; GONÇALVES, 2010).

Any and all complications and care provided to the patient will be attached and organized, and this information will be formally called a medical record, which will have its information restricted only to the healthcare professionals involved with the patient. They will also be used to control charges for materials and medical fees during the hospitalization period.

This document will contain all the anamnesis and progression of the pathology to which it refers, and will be protected by law, under penalty of loss and violation by third parties who are not from the health area, and will also have to be kept intact for a period of 20 years, and can only be destroyed after encryption, for the purpose of safeguarding them (ITO et al, 2011).

Decree Law No. 94.406 of June 8, 1987, which regulates Law No. 7.498 of June 25, 1996 in its Art. 14, emphasizes the obligation of all nursing staff to "record all nursing care activities in the patient's medical record" (BRASIL, 1996) and also through COFEN resolution 311/2007 approving the new reformulation of the code of ethics for nursing professionals, which states in Art. 68, the duty to "record in medical records and other documents specific to nursing, information relating to the process of caring for the person." (BRASIL, 2007).

The COREN/SP notes manual (2011) states that nursing notes must be recorded in the nursing report, which is an integral part of the medical record, so failing to record information on the procedures carried out could lead to future problems, both when it comes to collecting this data for the hospital's billing, and in legal proceedings that may be committed, and finally, the omission violates the professional code of ethics.

Another important issue is to maliciously write off or charge for materials, medicines or fees that are untrue or undue. Such practices violate the consumer protection code: according to Law No. 8078 of September 11, 1990, in art. 42 of the Sole Paragraph, the consumer who is charged an "undue amount" has the right to a refund equal to double the amount overpaid, plus monetary restatement. According to Article 42 of the Sole Paragraph of Law 8078/1990, consumers who are charged an "undue amount are entitled to a refund, for an amount equal to double what they paid in excess, plus monetary restatement and legal interest, except in the event of justifiable deception" (BRASIL, 1990).

Other ethical issues regarding nursing notes can be found in art. 42 of Law no. 8078 of 11/09/1990 (BRASIL, 1990), which prohibits professionals from signing nursing actions that they have not carried out, as well as allowing their actions to be signed by another professional. Furthermore, the use of correction pencils, erasers or crossed-out lines to hide the record is not allowed, due to its legal implications. The ethical issues surrounding nursing notes are fundamental to the practice of the profession and to the hospital economy, as unethical notes lead to lawsuits and denials by health insurance companies (COREN/SP, 2011).

Therefore, according to the COREN/SP manual (2011, p. 11), in order to make good, organized and quality notes, they must be:

a) They must be legitimate, complete, clear, concise, objective, punctual and chronological;

b) They must be preceded by the date and time, with the professional's signature and identification at the end of each record;

c) No erasures, interlineations, blank lines or spaces;

d) Contain observations made, care given, whether standardized, routine or specific;

e) They should also include the patient's responses to the care prescribed by the nurse, complications, signs and symptoms observed;

f) They should be recorded after the care has been provided, guidance given or information obtained;

g) They should prioritize the description of characteristics such as measured size (cm, mm, etc.), quantity (ml, l, etc.), color and shape;

h) Do not contain terms that give a connotation of value (good, bad, a lot, a little, etc.);

i) Only use abbreviations that are prescribed in the literature;

j) They should refer to simple data that does not require further scientific study. It is not correct, for example, for the nursing technician or assistant to write down data relating to the patient's physical examination, such as distended abdomen, tympanic; isochoric pupils, etc., since, in order to obtain this data, it is necessary to have carried out the previous physical examination, which is a private action of the nurse.

4.3 THE IMPORTANCE OF NOTES FOR HOSPITALS

The essence of modern hospitals is geared towards financial capital, and according to this, they are considered to be companies, with "economic activity". Within this context, we need to understand the role of the patient, who becomes a consumer and the hospital a service provider, both of whom are part of the legal framework, guided by laws and the code of ethics of their respective professional councils (OGUISSO, 2003).

According to Santos (2003, p.35), nursing "produces a lot of information on a daily basis that is inherent to patient care. It is possible to estimate that nursing is responsible for more than 50% of the information contained in patient records". In this sense, quality alone is not enough; quantitative information is also needed, such as: the quantity of masks, gloves, caps, slippers, medicines, etc. used. This fact leads private hospitals to generate their invoices relating to these costs, so nursing records are documents of clinical, legal and institutional importance (GALANTE, 2005).

In a hospital, the nursing team plays an important role, as it is the largest group of staff. The nurse has the competence to lead the nursing team, manage materials and, among other things, carry out nursing audits (CUNHA, 2006).

In addition, over time these records have taken on important characteristics and functions within institutions, becoming tools that facilitate the planning of nursing actions. Although legislation points to the importance of nursing records in order to document and support the profession, research shows that even though professionals are aware of these conditions, they still do not carry out nursing records with quality, or even consider them as a working tool, making it impossible for them to function (FERNANDES, 2010).

Therefore, note-taking should be valued, since it is one of the means of evaluating both the care provided to the client through the adoption of quality indicators for nursing care, and an administrative tool, and there is a positive correlation between records of expenses and billing and the quality of care provided.

4.4 PRONTUARIOS

The patient's medical record is a document that contains information about the patient, the illness and its treatment. It is kept when the patient visits a health service, is admitted to hospital or simply has a consultation.

There are reports of documents similar to medical records dating back to the stone age, with the surgical papyrus, acquired by Edwin Smith, being one of the oldest known documents, he acquired it and translated it, the document covered more than forty-eight clinical and surgical cases (ITO et al, 2011).

According to Possari (2005), the patient's medical record is an extremely important document, because it contains not only the anamnesis, but also all the assistance provided, an analysis of the progression of the disease and the results achieved.

Each patient's medical record should be individualized and contain their full identification, including gender, address, parents' names and place of birth.

According to Marin, Massad and Azevedo (2003), patient records have the following functions: To support the health care process by serving as a source of clinical and administrative information for decision-making and a means of communication shared between all the professionals who work in this process; It is the legal record of actions carried out by the multi-professional team; It should support research, clinical and epidemiological studies, quality assessment, among others: It should promote the teaching and management of services by providing data for billing and reimbursement, insurance authorization, support for organizational aspects and cost management.

4.5 ELECTRONIC MEDICAL RECORDS

With the frequent changes in health institutions, we are living in a new era, the era of computerized systems, which should be understood within the health area as an instrument to support the interventions carried out and recorded in the patient's medical record.

According to the Pan American Health Organization (2006), information technology aims to promote its application in user service, involving the creation, management and supply of fundamental technological resources for the development and operation of an organization's document systems.

ITO et al (2011), states that the electronic medical record is a means of storing clinical and administrative health information, with several benefits, such as: faster access to patient problems; Access to

up-to-date scientific knowledge; Improved decision-making; Effective patient care and cost reduction. With the electronic medical record, information can be obtained more quickly.

So, for Marin, Massad and Azevedo (2003), the basic purpose of the electronic medical record is to bring together all kinds of information produced in different ways, at different times, by different professionals in the healthcare team, with the aim of being an electronic structure for keeping information on the patient's state of health and care.

According to Lessa (2002), the main benefits of electronic medical records are: an increase in the quality of medical records; an improvement in the quality and completeness of data collection; a reduction in the amount of space needed to store information; an improvement in decision making; easier statistical research and research by professionals into information pertaining to procedures, among others.

Given all the purposes and benefits of electronic medical records, we have to bear in mind that they must be done in an agile and efficient manner, but always acting ethically and securely. In order to ensure this security, confidentiality, integrity and availability will be preserved so that we have the privacy of this data.

5 METHODOLOGY

5.1 TYPE OF STUDY

The study took a qualitative approach, i.e. one that considers that there is an inseparable link between the objective world and the subject's subjectivity that cannot be translated into numbers. The interpretation of phenomena and the attribution of meanings were basic to the qualitative research process (CHIZZOTTI, 2002).

It was also descriptive exploratory, as described by Clemente (2010), in which the aim is to provide the researcher with more knowledge about the topic or research problem.

Thus, this study is characterized as a case study, which for Chizzotti (2002, p.43), the case study collects and records data from "a particular case or several cases in order to organize an orderly and critical report of an experience or evaluate it analytically, with the aim of making decisions about it or proposing a transformative action."

5.2 RESEARCH SCENARIO

The study was carried out in a medical inpatient unit of a general private hospital, which treats patients from all specialties, both private and public.

5.3 SUBJECTS

5.3.1 Patient

The inclusion criteria were the records of patients hospitalized in the medical clinic, totaling 10 records, from one week to one month. Exclusion criteria were patients who had been hospitalized for more than a month and patients who had been readmitted.

5.3.2 Nurse

The inclusion criteria were to invite the five nurses responsible for the Medical Clinic, who work at all times, in order to facilitate access to and handling of patient records. Exclusion criteria were those who did not wish to take part in the study.

5.4 INSTRUMENT

A form was drawn up with a script on the following variables: patient profile (age, gender, occupation and clinical diagnosis), data on the object of the research (essential items for good nursing notes, according to the COREN/SP manual (2011) (APPENDIX C).

5.5 DATA COLLECTION

After presenting the research to the nurse and the patient, they were invited to take part, and once they had accepted, we asked them to sign the ICF, informing them that their identity would be preserved.

Patient records were selected according to the inclusion and exclusion criteria. The records were collected in August and September 2013 (according to schedule).

5.6 RESEARCH ETHICS

This study was evaluated by the Research Ethics Committee (CEP) and in accordance with the requirements of the Free and Informed Consent Form (TCLE), it was approved under opinion number 363.720 dated 14/08/2013, fulfilling the requirements of CNS resolution 196/96, which incorporates the four basic references of bioethics under the ethics of individuals and groups: autonomy, non-maleficence, beneficence and justice; thus assuring the participants of this research total secrecy and anonymity with regard to their identification and also the free right to participate or not in the research, being able to abandon it without any loss, being exempt from any payment or receipt of money for participating in this study.

5.7 RISKS AND BENEFITS

5.7.1 Risks

The research was not intended to harm or expose those involved, the patients' names were kept confidential, the data collection instruments will remain in the custody of students Abel dos Santos, Larissa N. Azevedo da Silva and Marcelo dos Santos Miranda for a period of 5 years, and will be incinerated after this period. It is considered that all research involving human beings involves risks, which have been minimized by keeping the patients' names anonymous, using "P" followed by numbers. Example: P1, P2,...

5.7.2 Benefits

To give professionals a clearer understanding of nursing notes and progression, showing them the importance of carrying out this activity with quality, in order to diagnose efficiently and be able to provide humanized and precise care.

5.8 DATA ANALYSIS

The data was analyzed using the content analysis method. Content analysis is a research methodology used to describe and interpret the content of all kinds of documents and texts pertinent to the subject being researched. It leads to systematic descriptions, whether qualitative or quantitative, as well as helping to reinterpret messages and reach an understanding of their meanings at a level that goes beyond ordinary reading (BARDIN, 1979).

6 Results and discussion

A qualitative assessment was made of 10 medical records of patients admitted to the medical clinic between August and September 2013. The profile of the patients in the records analyzed showed that nine patients were male and only one record of a female patient; however, this data is not in line with the results observed in the literature (ROCHEDO, 2010), where the predominance of cases in the medical clinic is female. This may be related to the size of the sample observed, which is smaller than the study carried out by Rochedo (2010).

With regard to age, the patients were between 30 and 94 years old. This data is in line with that found by Rochedo (2010) and Moreno (2009), who observed that the most recurrent cases in medical clinics are patients aged between 20 and over 80 years old.

Diagnoses of the following pathologies were found in the medical records: Liver Abscess (one case), Perianal Abscess (one case), Chagas Disease (one case), Pneumonia (one case), Polytrauma (one case), AIDS (Acquired Immunodeficiency Syndrome) (one case) and Stroke (Encephalic Vascular Accident), the latter being the most prevalent among the patients with four cases (TABLE 1).

Lachne et al (1999) and Rochedo (2010) also observed a higher frequency of cardiovascular pathologies in their studies. This fact is probably related to the high rate of cardiovascular problems in the world, such as strokes, which are considered one of the main causes of death in the world (CHAVES, 2000).

With regard to the stroke cases found in the study, it was observed that in all cases the patients were aged between 74 and 94 and were male. Pires (2004), in a study carried out in São Paulo, also observed that the majority of stroke cases were between 60 and 93 years of age, with a predominance of cases in male patients, and that smoking, alcoholism, heart disease, hypertension, diabetes mellitus and dyslipidemia were the most common risk factors. The profiles of the patients in the medical records analyzed are illustrated in Table 1.

Table 1- Profile of the patients in the medical records analyzed.

Patients	Age	Sex	Occupation	Clinical Diagnosis
P1	*77*	*M*	*Retired*	*AVE*
P2	*40*	*M*	*Self-employed*	*AIDS*
P3	*37*	*M*	*Nursing Technician*	*Chagas disease*
P4	*30*	*M*	*Student*	*Liver Abscess*
P5	*47*	*F*	*Housewife*	*Pneumonia*

P6	*74*	*M*	*Retired*	*AVE*
P7	*34*	*M*	*Broker*	*Polytraumatized*
P8	*84*	*M*	*Retired*	*AVE*
P9	*53*	*M*	*Professor*	*Perianal abscess*
P10	*94*	*M*	*Medical*	*AVE*

Source: Survey form (2013).

When analyzing the medical records, we divided them into two categories: those of a legal nature and those of a care nature, taking into account the items recommended by the COREN/SP manual (2011), which establishes essential items for making quality nursing notes.

The items that make up the category of legal character are: legible, clear and objective notes; the date, time, signature and identification of the professional; erasures, blank lines or spaces and only abbreviations provided for in the literature. The results observed for these items are illustrated in Graph 1.

Graph 1 - Results of the legal aspects analyzed in the medical records according to COREN/SP (2011).

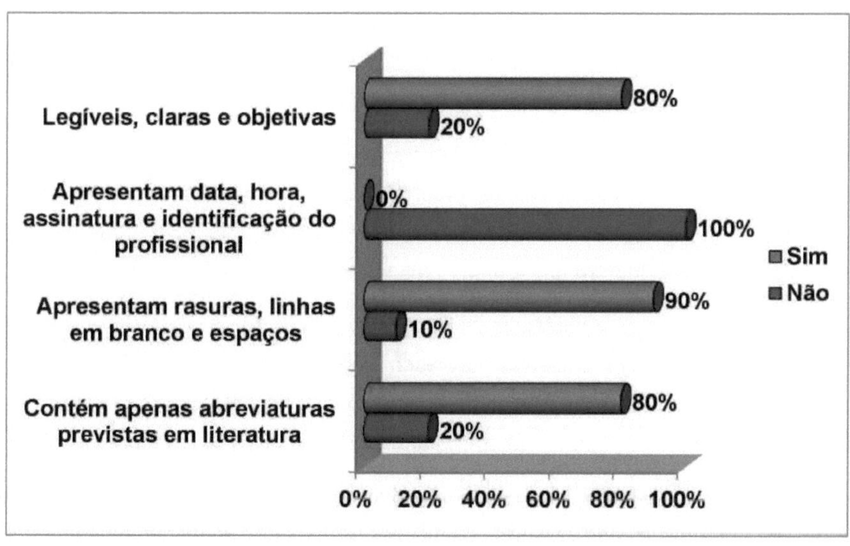

Source: Survey form (2013).

In this study, it was observed that 80% of the notes were legitimate, clear and objective, which is a positive point, since clear and objective notes provide a better understanding for anyone reading the medical record of what happened to the patient during a given period (POTTER, 2012).

The data analyzed was very similar to that found in a study carried out by Luz (2007), who analyzed 144 medical records in three hospital inpatient units of a private health plan, where he observed that around 50% to 70% of the nursing notes were legitimate and clear.

Ochoa-Vigo (2001) also observed that more than 70% of the notes are legible and clear.

Legible handwriting facilitates the work of the health team, so that the information written down is not misinterpreted, which can bring risks to the patient, and can also involve both legal aspects and health audits (POTTER, 2012).

100% of the medical records analyzed did not contain any of the following items: date, time, signature or identification of the professional, with the lack of date and time being the most recurrent factors in the notes. A similar result was found by Luz (2007).

Notes without dates and times should not be kept, as the chronology of events with the patient is fundamental for continuity of care and predictability of possible complications (LUZ, 2007).

It is important to remember that it is essential to record the date and time of the procedures carried out in the medical records, as they are valuable documents for research, teaching, audits, evaluation of care and legal issues. In this sense, it should be noted that access to medical records is a patient's right (OCHOA-VIGO, 2001).

A few medical records lacked the signature and stamp of the responsible professional. However, this is not in line with what has been observed in the literature. LUZ (2007) observed, in his study carried out in three health units in Curitiba, that most of the medical records did not have the signature and stamp of the professional responsible for the entry.

The Federal Nursing Council (COFEN) - in its Resolution 191/96 (BRASIL, 1996) stipulates that nursing staff must identify themselves after each record using their name, category and COREN/SP registration number, as well as the professional's stamp. However, in the notes observed, there was a lack of use of the stamp and signature. This is probably due to the professionals' lack of habit of using the stamp.

In addition, 90% of the cases had erasures, blank lines and spaces. In the case of erasures and errors, corrections should be made using the terms "I say" or "Correction", and then write down what is correct, and then continue with the record (LUZ, 2007), who found similar results in his research, with regard to erasures and errors, as well as corrections of the respective errors. However, Ochoa-Vigo (2001) found a low percentage of errors and erasures in nursing notes.

In 80% of cases, the notes did not deviate from the standard, containing only abbreviations provided for in the literature, which means that the notes are interpreted correctly, without duplicating information.

Valderrama (2009), in his study, observed that the use of non-standardized acronyms accounted for around 40% of all notes taken by nursing technicians, which is twice as much as was found in the study in question. This also shows a lack of standardization in the notes taken in Brazil, despite current legislation.

The items that make up the care category include: observations made and care provided, patients' responses to the care prescribed by the nurse, guidance provided or information obtained, priority is given to descriptions of characteristics, measured size, quantity, color and shape, terms that give a connotation of value and simple data without further scientific study. The results observed for these items are illustrated in Graph 2.

Graph 2 - Identification of data on care parameters in medical records.

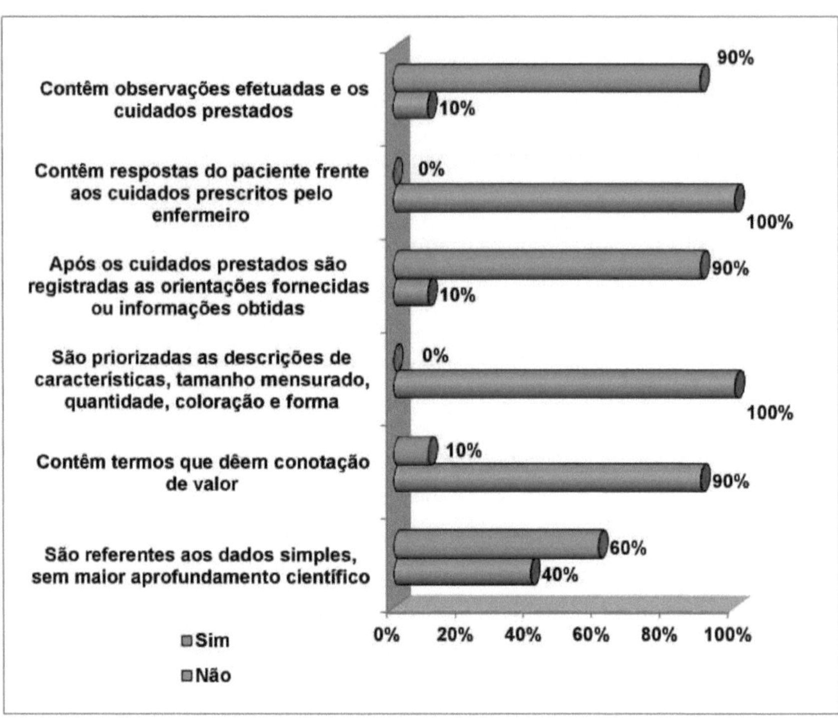

Source: Survey form (2013).

In this category it was identified that 90% of the medical records contained the care provided, and 100% of the notes did not contain the patient's responses to the care prescribed by the nurse or the signs and symptoms observed.

Bresolin (2013) observed that around 40% of nursing notes were missing descriptions of the care provided and checks, and that 11% of the records were incomplete. However, the result observed in our study was different to that found by BRESOLIN (2013).

With regard to the lack of response from patients to the care provided, Ochoa-Vigo (2001) also observed that the rate of information obtained by patients is generally very low. However, it was hoped to find more of this type of information. Patients' ideas should be better described, as well as their feelings and perspectives on the disease. This information should always be accompanied by clinical data in order to help guide nursing interventions (OCHOA-VIGO, 2001).

Studies by Angerami (1976) already showed that nursing does not pay enough attention to the subjective aspects of patients, as there is little information describing their psychospiritual and psychosocial conditions, and Fâvero (1979) proposed, back then, that this trend in nursing is related to the model used in many nursing schools, which show a lack of teaching of the psychosocial aspects that are so fundamental in health care.

Of the professionals who reported on the care provided, in 90% of cases there were records of the guidance and information provided after the care. It is worth noting that the lack of information on care and guidance can be used as evidence of poor professional behavior or low-quality care, meaning that another professional reading the medical record will not be able to determine whether the patient was adequately cared for (POTTER 2012).

All the notes did not prioritize the description of characteristics such as: measured size, quantity, color and shape. This is a very negative point found in the notes of the institution analyzed, because the use of exact measurement establishes the accuracy of the facts, being decisive for possible changes in the patient's condition (POTTER 2012).

In the study carried out by Luz (2007), the absence of descriptions of the characteristics presented by the patients was also observed. These measurements are very important for assessing body function and responses to treatment, and should contain all possible parameters.

It was also observed that around 90% of the notes did not contain terms that gave a connotation of value and 60% of the notes referred to simple data without going into greater scientific detail. This fact was also observed by Valderrama (2009), who noted that 41% of the nursing technicians did not make a simple report and went into greater depth in their notes, which is considered inappropriate in a note-taking process, because for greater scientific depth, a prior physical examination is required, which is a private function of the nurse.

Finally, it can be said that nursing notes are important and essential for assessing the quality of the nursing care provided, as well as providing data on the patient's progress. Thus, the more and better the nursing team records their actions, the more their work will be valued, as well as helping to ensure the continuity of the patient's treatment.

Therefore, the entry in a patient's medical record is not only an act of registration, but also a legal act, as it refers to the data necessary for legal proof.

However, the results of this study show that there is a lack of information on actions and their characteristics. It would therefore be necessary to continue the study in healthcare institutions in order to more reliably measure the limitations of data in medical records, held by all the professionals who have access to it. This could be a strategy to significantly improve record-keeping, guaranteeing quality of care and better management of services.

7 FINAL CONSIDERATIONS

It is considered that:

- The nursing records presented were inaccurately correct in terms of lack of date and time of the notes, signature and identification of the professional, and with erasures, blank lines and unfilled spaces and lack of patient information about the care provided.

- The standardization of nursing records (notes and progress) is an important factor in monitoring the patient's progress.

- Nursing notes still need to be reviewed in order to obtain better documentation of the care provided to the patient, as well as to identify the problems detected that will help to intervene and meet their needs.

- There is a need for a continuing education program for nurses and the entire nursing team because, in addition to providing quality patient care, it will promote professional development and thus better define the nurse's role in the nursing team.

REFERENCES

ANGERAMI E.L.S, MENDES I.A.C, PEDRAZZANI J.C. Critical analysis of nursing notes. **Rev Bras Enferm,** v.29, n.3, p. 28-37. 1976.

BARDIN, L. **Content analysis**. Sâo Paulo: Atlas**, 1979.**

BRAZIL. Federal Nursing Council. **Resolution N. 311, of February 8, 2007.** Approves the reformulation of the code of ethics for nursing professionals. Available at:

<http://www.portalcofen.gov.br/site/2007/materais.asp?article iD=7221§ioniD=34/>. Accessed on: 17 Apr. 2013.

. Ministry of Health. Pan American Health Organization. **Development of health systems and services**: Brazil's regulatory policy: Technical Series. Brasilia (DF), 2006. Available at: <http//www.opas.org.br/serviço/arquivos/sala5571.pdf>. Accessed on: 17 Apr. 2013.

. Presidency of the Republic. **Decree Law No. 94.406, of June 8, 1987.** Regulates Law 7.498, of June 25, 1996. Available at: < http://novo.portalcofen.gov.br/decreto-n-9440687_4173.html>. Accessed on: 17 Apr. 2013.

. **Law No. 8078, of September 11, 1990**. Provides for consumer protection and other measures. Available at: <http://www.planalto.gov.br/ccivil 03/leis/l8078.htm>. Accessed on: April 17, 2013.

BRESOLiN, P.; FAVERi, F. Occurrence of failures in nursing notes in a clinical hospitalization unit. **Revista Eletrônica Gestao & Saùde**, v.4, n. 3, p.1235-41. 2013.

CARRiJO, A.R.; OGUiSSO, T. Trajectory of Nursing Notes: a survey in national journals (1957-2005). **Rev Bras Enferm**. Sâo Paulo, n. 59, p. 454-458. 2006. Ed. esp.

CIANCIARRULO, T.1. **Basic instruments for care:** a challenge for the quality of care. Sâo Paulo (SP): Atheneu, 1996.

CHAVES, M. L. F. Cerebrovascular accident: conceptualization and risk factors. **Rev Bras Hipertens.** v.4, p.372-82, 2000.

CHIZZOTTI, A. **Pesquisa em ciências humanas e sociais.** 5. ed. Sao Paulo: Cortez, 2002.

CLEMENTE, F. **Qualitative, exploratory and phenomenological research:** some basic concepts. 2010. Available at: <http://www.administradores.com.br/informe-se/artigos/pesquisa-qualitativa- exploratory-and-phenomenological-some-basic-concepts/14316/>. Accessed on: 17 Apr. 2013.

REGIONAL NURSING COUNCIL OF SAO PAULO - COREN-SP. **Nursing notes manual,** 2011. Sao Paulo: Coren-SP, 2011. 11 p.

CUNHA, I.C.K.o.; XIMENEs NETo, F.R.G. Competências Gerenciais de enfermeiras: Um novo velho Desafio? **Texto Contexto enfer.**, Florianópolis, v. 15, n. 3, jul./sep. 2006. Available at: <http://redalyc.uaemex.mx/redalyc/pdf/714/71415313.pdf>. Accessed on: September 29, 2013.

DANIEL, L.F. **Atitudes interpessoais em enfermagem**. Sao Paulo: EPU, 1983.

DIAS, D.C., SILVA, M.J.P. The record of nursing practice: from the reality of routine care to the utopia of individualized care. **Rev. Nursing**. v.11, n.2, p.2166. 1999.

D"INNOCENZO, M. et al. **Indicators, audits, certifications**: quality tools for health management. Sao Paulo: Martinar, 2006.

FÂVERO N. **Study of nursing notes in direct patient care**. 98 f. 1979. Thesis (Dissertaçao) - University of Sao Paulo. Ribeirao Preto Nursing School, 1979.

FERNANDES, A. P. et al. Quality of nursing notes related to cardiopulmonary resuscitation compared to the Utstein model. **Acta paul. enferm.**, Sao Paulo , v. 23, n. 6, 2010 . Available at: <http://www.scielo.br/scielo.php?script=sci_arttext&pid=S0103-21002010000600007&lng=en&nrm=iso>. Accessed on: October 16, 2013.

GALANTE, A.C. **Nursing reports as quality indicators.** Brasilia, DF: Gama Filho University; UNIMED University, 2005. Available at: <http://www.fundacaounimed.org.br/site/Monografias>. Accessed on: September 25, 2013.

HORTA, W.A. Dos instrumentos básicos de enfermagem. **Rev. Esc Enferm USP**. p.3-4.1970.

ITO, E.E. et al. **Nursing notes: a** reflection of care. Sao Paulo (SP): Martinari, 2011. p.5-7.

LACHNE, M. et al. Profile of patients in the Medical Clinic outpatient clinic. **Rev Med Hosp Sao Vicente de Paulo**, v.11, p.27-29, 1999.

LESSA, M.C. et al. Communication in nursing: modernization of the hospital information system: the use of electronic medical records . In: BRAZILIAN SYMPOSIUM ON NURSING COMMUNICATION, 8., 2002, Ribeirao

Preto(SP). **Anais...** Ribeirao Preto School of Nursing, 2002. Available at: <http://www.proceedings.scielo.br/scielo.php?pid=MSC0000000052002000200038& script=sci_arttext>. Accessed on: April 17, 2013.

LOURENÇO, M.R. et al. Analysis of nursing notes according to dugas. In: SIMPÒSIO BRASILEIRO DE COMUNICAÇÃO EM ENFERMAGEM, 7., 2000,

Ribeirao Preto (SP). **Proceedings...** Ribeirao Preto (SP). Ribeirao Preto School of Nursing, 2000. p. 37-41.

LUZ, A.; MARTINS, A.P.; DYNEWICZ, A.M. Caracteristicas de anotações de enfermagem encontrados em auditoria. **Revista Eletrônica de Enfermagem**. v.9, n.2, p 344-361, May/Aug. 2007. Available at:

<http://www.fen.ufg.br/revista/v9/n2/v9n2a05.htm> Accessed on: 15 Oct. 2013.

MARIN, H.F.; MASSAD, E.; AZEVEDO, N.R.S. Evaluation of the information recorded in the medical records of patients admitted to an obstetric ward. **Acta Paul Enferm**. p. 7-13. 2003;

MATOS, S.S. **Written communication of nursing actions:** a contribution to undergraduate teaching. 130 f. 1997. Master's degree dissertation. Belo Horizonte: School of Nursing, Federal University of Minas Gerais, 1997.

MATSUDA L.M. et al. Nursing notes/records: a communication tool for quality care. **Rev Eletrônica Enferm.**; v.8, n.3, p. 415-21. 2006. Available at:

<http://www.fen.ufg.br/revista/revista8_3/v8n3a12.htm>. Accessed on: 17 Apr. 2013.

MORENO, A.C. et al. Socio-demographic profile of out-patient clinic first assessment. **Eur**

Psychiatry J, p. 24. 2009.

NÒBREGA, M.R.S. On the subject of nursing notes. **Enfermagem Atual**, v.2, n.11, p.30-1.1980.

OCHOA-VIGO, K. et al. Evaluation of the quality of nursing notes based on the nursing process. **Rev Esc Enferm USP**. Sao Paulo, v.35, n.4, p.390-98. 2001.

OGUISSO, T. **Os aspectos legais da anotação de enfermagem no prontàrio do paciente [The legal aspects of nursing notes in the patient's medical record** [livre-docência]. Rio de Janeiro (RJ): Ana Néri Nursing School, 1975.

. Ethical and legal dimensions of nursing notes in patient records. **Rev Paul Enferm**. p. 245-254, 2003.

PIRES, S. L.; GAGLIARDI, R. J.; GORZONI, M. L. Study of the frequencies of the main risk factors for ischemic stroke in the elderly. **Arq Neuropsiquiatr**. p. 844-51. 2004.

POSSARI, J.F. **Patient records and nursing records**. Sâo Paulo: Latria, 2005.

POTTER, P. A.; PERRY, A.G. **Fundamentals of nursing**. 7. ed.

Janeiro: Elsevier, 2012. V.1.

ROCHEDO, M.P.R.R.; GUEDES, M.A.B. Profile of patients at the outpatient medical clinic. Preliminary study. **Rev Bras Clin Med**, Rio de Janeiro, v.8, p.33-6. 2010

SANTOS, S.R; PAULA, A.F.A; LIMA, J.P. O enfermeiro e sua percepção sobre o sistema manual de registro no prontàrio. **Rev Latino am Enferm**. v.11, n.1, p.80-7, 2003.

TONG, P.; GONÇALVES, S.E.F. **Communication in the systematization of perioperative nursing care as a reference for quality in service.** Communication and Health. Latin American Association of Communication Researchers. làcomunicacion . 2010. Available Available at:

<http://www.alaic.net/VII_congresso/gt/gt_10/GT_6.html>. Accessed on: 17 Apr. 2013.

VALDERRAMA, M.C.S.; CAMPOS, O. Concurrent nursing audit in an intensive care unit. **Boletim de enfermagem**, Paranà, v. 3, n. 2, p. 73-87. 2009.

VENTURINE, D.A; MARCON, S.S. Nursing notes in a surgical unit of a teaching hospital. **Rev Bras Enferm**, v. 61, n. 5, p. 570-577, 2008.

CHAPTER II - MEDICATION INTERACTION: NURSES' KNOWLEDGE AND PRACTICE.

CLAYSE JENNIFER ALVES DE SOUZA MARIA TITA PORTAL SACRAMENTO MARCELO WILLIAMS OLIVEIRA DE SOUZA MARIA LUCIA RIBEIRO

SUMMARY

The administration of medication is a practice that requires constant updating and a great deal of attention. In health institutions, the nursing team is responsible for this process, so nurses must have knowledge of the subject in order to detect early the possible risks and complications caused by drug therapy, taking into account the characteristics of the drugs and especially the possibilities of drug interactions. The aim of this study was to analyze nurses' knowledge and practice of drug interactions. We opted for a methodology with a descriptive qualitative approach and conducted the study with 20 nurses from a private hospital located in the metropolitan region of Belém.

Results: Approximately 50% of the nurses are aware of the action and reaction of the drugs and approximately 50% are unaware of the side effects. The conclusion is that there is a need for training on the subject.

Key words: Medicines, drug interactions, nurses.

1. INTRODUCTION

In Brazil, the administration of medicines is a daily activity that is the legal responsibility of the nursing team, in accordance with Law No. 7.498/86 (which regulates the practice of nursing and makes other provisions), Decree No. 94.406/87, in all health institutions and is therefore of great importance for both the professional category and the clients. The administration of medicines is a complex process that occupies a considerable place in the health system for the treatment of illnesses, and for many the alternative to the search for a cure is the use of medicines.

The nursing team is responsible for administering medication, observing the basic principles in order to ensure the client's safety, thereby guaranteeing good care. This process requires a great deal of attention and constant updating on the part of these professionals.

In order to administer a drug safely and efficiently, nurses must know the drug's action on the body, methods and routes of administration and elimination, side reactions, maximum and therapeutic dose, toxic effects, as well as knowledge of the administration technique and the client. In order to guarantee safety in the administration of medicines, the *five rights* were created, which are measures used to minimize these possible errors. They are: the right drug, the right client, the right dose, the right route of administration and the right time (MIASSO; CASSIANI, 2000). Currently, nine observation measures are used, i.e. the *right nine.* The following must be observed: right patient, right drug, right route of administration, right dose, right time, right documentation, right action, right form, right response.

These requirements are not present in the vast majority of health institutions. As the nurse responsible for the nursing team, he/she has a responsibility in this work process in which the administration of medicines is routinely delegated, being at a supervisory level and although he/she is not responsible for prescribing the medicine, he/she must know all the aspects and phases involved in administering it, in order to prevent errors and mistakes that harm the client.

It should be emphasized that such observations and evaluations can only be made if these professional nurses have mastery and knowledge of the action of the drugs administered, i.e. the greater the nurse's knowledge of the subject, the greater their ability to carry out this activity. However, day-to-day practice points to a different reality, as professionals don't always have sufficient knowledge to take on this responsibility.

During drug therapy, the client should be systematically observed and assessed for possible unwanted reactions, as well as the possibility of drug interactions, in order to reduce the possible risks. The term drug interactions refers to the interference of one drug in the action of another or of a food or nutrient in the action of medicines (TRATO, 1999).

With constant scientific and technological growth, new drugs are appearing, expanding the clinical practice of polypharmacy, i.e. the practice of combining drugs and thus increasing the capacity of professionals to meet the demands of clients in morbid processes, whether in hospital or at home, bringing with them benefits in therapeutic treatments, but also the risk of drug interactions, which deserve special attention; Bearing in mind that medicines are made up of chemical substances which can interact/react with each other, resulting in toxic products for the body, and with all the responsibility associated with this, it is one of the most important aspects for teaching nursing care.

It is essential for nurses to reflect on the execution of medical prescriptions, which are invariably carried out according to pre-established schedules in almost all healthcare institutions. And, according to Mengardo and Oguisso (1986), it is "like a system of functional distribution of tasks" for the nursing team, thus not taking into account the characteristics of the drugs and especially the possibilities of drug interactions. Most of the literature on the subject is aimed at doctors and pharmacists, with little or no discussion of the role of nurses in this area. This reflection should be implemented and encouraged in undergraduate courses, so that nursing students are aware of the importance of knowledge and practice in pharmacology and its implications for effective client care. According to Potter and Perry (2001) nurses are responsible for knowing the effects of a drug, administering it correctly, controlling the client's response and helping them to self-administer it.

This study will serve to disseminate, promote and expand knowledge on the subject so that nurses can acquire an appropriate basis, and it is essential that they systematically supervise and assess clients for possible drug interactions.

1.1 BACKGROUND

In my academic life, I have seen how difficult it is for nurses to talk about drug interactions, because some hospital departments have a very large volume of drugs that are almost always administered at the same times. It is not possible to identify whether this deficiency lies in the academic training of these professionals or in the lack of a search for knowledge as professionals.

The curricular matrix of the nursing course includes the subject of Pharmacology, which is of fundamental importance to the training of professional nurses. However, this subject is not given due importance by academics and may not be sufficient for professional practice, and the relationship between theory and practice may be unsatisfactory and this conception will reflect in the little knowledge of these future professionals in relation to drug interactions.

It is believed that by knowing these elements, nurses can carry out their daily work and intervene in the medication routine in order to prevent the occurrence of adverse reactions resulting from drug interactions.

Based on the findings, it can be seen that little is known about the subject and that drug interactions are part of the day-to-day routine of the nursing team in healthcare institutions. Nurses are responsible for formulating and organizing how and when prescribed medications should be administered, often done randomly, with little or no knowledge of the subject.

Professionals must know the necessary actions regarding a patient's medication, so that they can carry out their role with safety, awareness, responsibility and efficiency (SILVA, 2003). It is therefore essential for nurses to have a broad view of the medication system and each of its processes, in order to avoid possible errors that could result in harm to the client.

Drug interactions that do occur, usually occasionally, tend to increase the length of hospitalization, increase the cost of treatment and cause greater morbidity for the client.

In order to prevent future problems, it is necessary to adopt educational measures for the nursing team involved in administering medication as an important factor in preventing possible medication errors.

Based on this reality, the question arises:

- How much do nurses know about drug interactions?
- What difficulties are encountered in nursing practice in relation to drug interactions?
- What do nurses need to know about drug interactions?

1.2 OBJECTIVES

General

- To analyze nurses' knowledge and practice of drug interactions.

Specifics

- To discuss nurses' knowledge and practice of drug interactions.
- To identify the difficulties encountered by nurses in their day-to-day knowledge and practice of drug interactions.
- To see if nurses are aware of adverse reactions resulting from drug interactions.

2. THEORETICAL FRAMEWORK

2.1 THE DIMENSIONING OF NURSING PRACTICE AND CLIENT SAFETY

Nursing is the largest professional category in the health sector in the world. In Brazil, it is estimated that nursing makes up more than 50% of the health workforce, controlling and carrying out most of the direct care provided to patients (MADUREIRA, et. al. 2000).

It is characterized as a profession in development in the country, both in terms of quantity and quality of professional practice. One of the aspects to consider in Brazilian nursing practice is the proportion of middle-level professionals, which is still much higher than that of higher-level professionals, so it can be seen that a large part of nursing actions are carried out by nursing assistants or technicians, who have technical knowledge and skills that allow them to carry out less complex practical activities, because they don't have the scientific knowledge to support the planning and decisions needed to implement nursing care, so they have to follow guidelines, prescriptions and carry out all the functions under the direct supervision of the nurse (HARADA, et. al. 2007). al. 2007).

Nurses are higher education professionals who have taken a degree course, with a variety of content that underpins health care for protection, promotion, recovery and rehabilitation in the various life cycles of human beings.

The development of more complex care activities must be carried out exclusively by nurses who, in addition to developing them, must plan and supervise them.

The excess of duties and activities of nurses not directly linked to nursing care can predispose to poor quality nursing care, since the overload of work and responsibilities of nurses means that these activities are not carried out as planned, and failure to improve and care carried out mechanically can cause possible risks to client safety.

Interactions are among the most important errors identified in drug prescriptions and are a cause for concern due to their ability to nullify the desired response or superimpose adverse effects on the disease, occurring with a frequency directly proportional to the complexity of the prescription. The iatrogenic potential of prescriptions stems from errors in the choice of dose, route of administration, frequency or drug interaction.

2.2 DRUG INTERACTIONS

Drug interactions are special types of pharmacological responses in which the effects of one or more drugs are altered by the simultaneous or previous administration of others, or by concurrent administration with food (OGA; BASILE, 1994). According to Thompson (1979), responses resulting from interaction can lead to a potentiation of the therapeutic effect, a reduction in efficacy, the appearance of adverse reactions with varying degrees of severity or even no change in the desired effect of the drug. Therefore, interactions between drugs can be useful (beneficial) or cause unfavorable responses not foreseen in the therapeutic regimen (adverse), or even be of little clinical significance.

Beneficial interactions are aimed at treating concomitant diseases, prolonging the duration of the effect, preventing or delaying the emergence of bacterial resistance and achieving a good outcome to the drug treatment, which are fundamental therapeutic approaches in various pathologies. The simultaneous prescription of several drugs and their subsequent administration is a common practice in classic therapeutic regimens, with the aim of improving the effectiveness of drugs, reducing toxicity or treating co-existing diseases. In the treatment of severe hypertension, for example, the combination of drugs with different mechanisms of action promotes the most efficient reduction in blood pressure (BOECHAT, 1991).

Along with the advantages of therapeutic possibilities comes the risk of unwanted effects and drug interactions. These undesirable interactions are those that lead to a reduction in the effect or a result contrary to expectations, an increase in the incidence of adverse effects and in the cost of therapy. These interactions result in a reduction in the drug's activity and consequently a loss of efficacy, are difficult to detect and may be responsible for the failure of therapy or the progression of the disease (HUSSAR, 2000).

Some factors related to the use of medicines, such as multiple pharmacological effects, multiple prescriptions, the client's lack of understanding of the pharmacological treatment, abuse of medicines, lack of information on the part of prescribers and dispensers and the use of medicines by self-medication, contribute to the occurrence of drug interactions, leading to therapeutic ineffectiveness and putting the client's life at risk.

In addition to the countless possibilities of interference between drugs, factors related to the individual (age, genetic makeup, physical and pathological state, nutritional status, type of diet) and the administration of the drug (dose, route, interval and sequence of administration) influence the response to treatment.

Interactions can be avoided if preventive measures are taken.

2.3 Mechanisms of drug interactions

Medicines can interact during preparation; at the time of absorption, distribution, metabolization, elimination or when binding to the pharmacological receptor. Thus, the mechanisms involved in this interactive process are classified according to the type of pharmacological phase in which they occur (GRAHAME-sMiTH; ARoNsoN,1988).

2.3.1 Pharmaceutical Interaction

These are physico-chemical interactions that occur when two or more drugs are administered in the same solution or mixed in the same container and are capable of making clinical therapy unfeasible. Therefore, they occur outside the body, during the preparation and administration of parenteral drugs and often result in precipitation or clouding of the solution; a change in the color of the drug or inactivation of the active ingredient (EisENBERG, 1997).

It is routine and customary for nurses to administer many drugs at the same time and to combine substances in the same solution or container, infused by multiple route devices (Y-shaped extensions). Thus, in this particular type of interaction, the nursing team plays an important role and can even prevent these situations, avoiding and minimizing undesirable occurrences during the procedure (SECOLI, 2001).

In everyday life, drugs that require continuous infusion are the most susceptible to pharmaceutical interactions, especially when they are administered concomitantly with other agents in single line venous catheters.

2.3.2 Pharmacokinetic Interaction

These interactions interfere with the pharmacokinetic profile of the drug and can affect the pattern of absorption, distribution, metabolization or excretion. These interactions are difficult to predict because they occur with drugs with unrelated active ingredients. They modify the magnitude and duration of the effect, but the final response of the drug is preserved (SECOLI, 2001).

Interactions that modify absorption involve the transfer of the drug from the site of administration to the bloodstream. Factors such as blood flow in the gastrointestinal tract (GIT), pH, motility, diet and the presence of other substances and the type of pharmaceutical formulation interfere in this event (CAMPOS; BARDINA, 1990). Some drugs that inhibit GI motility tend to reduce absorption, while the administration of other drugs alters pH and increases absorption. Delayed drug absorption can be an undesirable clinical situation, especially in the presence of acute symptoms such as pain. In interactions that affect the distribution pattern, the drug moves from the systemic circulation to the tissues.

This phase depends on the apparent volume of distribution and the binding fraction of the drugs to plasma proteins. Medicines have a high affinity for plasma proteins when associated with others, and can act as displacers and increase the serum concentration of the latter, leading to clinical manifestations that are not always beneficial (SECOLI, 2001).

In the process of metabolization, drugs are transformed by enzymes. The interactions that occur during this phase are precipitated by drugs that are able to inhibit or induce the enzyme system, leading to a delay in the biotransformation of the drug itself and others that have been administered simultaneously. The consequence of this delay is a longer pharmacological action time for the agent(s).

Interactions that modify excretion Most drugs are eliminated almost entirely by the kidneys. In this way, the rate of excretion of various agents can be modified by interactions along the nephron. Changes in urinary pH interfere with the degree of ionization of bases and weak acids, affecting pharmacological responses. The competition of drugs in the proximal tubule for tubular secretion is another mechanism used as a pharmacological strategy to prolong the action time of drugs (SECOLI, 2001).

2.3.4 Pharmacodynamic Interaction

Pharmacodynamic interaction causes a change in the biochemical or physiological effect of the drug. It usually occurs at the site of action of the drugs or through specific biochemical mechanisms, and is capable of causing similar (synergism) or opposite (antagonism) effects (FONSECA, 1994).

Synergism is a type of pharmacological response obtained from the combination of two or more drugs, the result of which is greater than the simple sum of the isolated effects of each one. It can occur with drugs that have the same mechanisms of action (additive); that act in different ways (summation) or with those that act on different pharmacological receptors (potentiation). Synergistic associations can have therapeutic or toxic effects, but their aim is to maximize therapeutic efficacy (NIES; SPIELBERG, 1996).

In antagonism, the pharmacological response of one drug is suppressed or reduced in the presence of another. An antagonist is therefore a drug that reduces or cancels out the effect of another and in pharmacological antagonism this event occurs at the level of receptors, i.e. the antagonist hinders the formation of the agonist-receptor complex.

Pharmacological antagonism can occur competitively when the antagonist competes with the agonist for the same receptor sites, non-competitively when the antagonist can bind to different sites or to the same binding site as the active drug, but does not compete with it but inactivates the receptor in such a way as to prevent the effective combination of the agonist. There is also partial antagonism or competitive dualism when two drugs with different intrinsic activities exert their actions on the same receptor site (CORBETT, 1982).

2.4 CLASSIFICATION OF POTENTIALLY INTERACTIVE DRUGS

The knowledge of drugs and the mastery of their therapeutic and toxic properties have transformed the use of pharmacology over the centuries. Drugs have gradually gained in importance. They have been used in various therapeutic studies with the aim of benefiting human beings. Considering that the word drug is defined in its broad sense as any chemical agent that affects life processes (ASPERHEIM, 1992).

In practice, therapeutic decisions rarely see drug interactions as an iatrogenic factor or responsible for ineffectiveness. In fact, this concern tends to be, on a day-to-day basis, more of a complicating agent than a facilitating one, so the literature shows that it is possible to predict which classes or drugs are potentially interactive (COSTA, 1984), to help doctors in the difficult task of prescribing and nurses in carrying out the proposed administration.

This activity doesn't just cover the act of administering drug therapy, it is seen as a process that includes several interrelated phases and includes requesting, distributing, following the medical prescription, interpreting this prescription, preparing the drugs and the actual administration, carried out by the nursing team. Added to these aspects is the assessment of the clinical response presented by the client. Precipitating drugs are able to move other agents away from their original site of action and thus affect the desired pharmacological effect. This group includes enzyme inducers and inhibitors, those that are highly bound to plasma proteins and those that alter kidney function.

Target or object drugs are those which, when they undergo a change in dose (even a small one), bring about a major change in effect. In these cases, the interaction often results in a reduction in the therapeutic efficacy of the drug used. However, for those drugs with a narrow therapeutic index, interactions lead to an increase in toxicity.

2.5 FACTORS RELATED TO THE ADMINISTRATION OF DRUGS THAT MAY LEAD TO AN INTERACTION

One of the factors that can lead to drug interactions is how the drug is administered. There are several factors, including:

Route of administration: some interactions are only possible when the two drugs are administered by the same route, such as orally, because the two or more drugs will be in contact for longer, increasing the chance of interactions occurring. Thus, if these drugs are administered by different routes, the possibility of interaction is reduced.

Time of administration: a short interval between the administration of one drug and another can increase the possibility of interaction, so knowing about interactions between drugs in advance allows you to choose the time of administration in order to reduce the occurrence of adverse interactions as much as possible.

Preparation for administration: interactions can start from the moment the drug is prepared. You need to pay attention to the correct diluent and the volume of infusion so as not to inactivate or potentiate the drug. Don't prepare the medication too many hours in advance, as this can make the job easier, but it can also compromise the stability of the medication.

Full treatment time: many of the interaction reactions only appear after some time of treatment, and it can take from a few hours to several weeks for them to occur.

Dosage: many interactions are dose-dependent, i.e. the higher the dose of the drugs involved, the greater the possibility of interaction. However, this may be different for potent drugs, such as those used in cancer treatment, where even small doses can lead to interactions.

Presentation: the form in which the drug is presented (liquid, tablets, lozenges, gradual release) can influence the possibility of interaction. For example, gradual-release drugs remain present in the body for longer and can therefore interact with other drugs that the client ingests.

2.6 RISK GROUPS

In practice, all individuals undergoing pharmacological therapy with two or more drugs are exposed to the effects of drug interactions, but some groups are certainly more susceptible, for example, the elderly, children, people with chronic diseases, users of intravenous drug infusion devices or enteral tubes (SECOLI, 2001).

In the elderly, the degeneration of organic systems, the excess of drugs prescribed, the length of treatment, the practice of self-medication and the numerous disorders of organs or systems responsible for the pharmacokinetics of drugs are some of the items that increase the possibility of adverse interactions (BOECHAT, 1991).

In children, we have to watch out for adverse reactions, such as allergic processes, which most often occur at this stage. According to the dosage, observe its volume and dilution according to the age group, where it is very different from the adult, in smaller quantities and much more diluted due to the capacity of their organism. Observe the intramuscular route of administration where the vastus lateralis (thigh) is recommended for children, as this muscle has the greatest volume capacity.

People with chronic diseases such as heart disease, liver disease, nephropathy; those with conditions affecting the immune system such as cancer, acquired immunodeficiency syndrome, lupus, rheumatoid arthritis or those undergoing therapy with immunosuppressive agents (corticosteroids, antineoplastic chemotherapy, biological response modifiers, among others) are exposed to treatment protocols with multiple drugs and for prolonged periods of time, important factors which, when combined, can precipitate undesirable reactions and aggravate the pathophysiological condition already in place.

Users of central venous catheters and enteral feeding tubes often suffer from digestive system disorders that can affect the movement and use of drug molecules in the body.

The maceration of tablets or sachets as a way of administering drugs through the enteral tube can facilitate the association of agents that are not compatible with each other, causing unwanted reactions. In addition, the nutrients in the diet can interfere with the action of the medication and cause harm to the client.

In intensive care unit clients, the continuous infusion of vasoactive drugs and the intermittent administration of others (antibiotics, analgesics, anxiolytics, antiemetics) are common and necessary; on the other hand, they are potential situations for the occurrence of adverse interactions, especially when care is not taken with regard to the compatibility of the drugs and the administration intervals between them (EISENBERG, 1997).

Nurses need to be aware of these very common risk situations, which often go unnoticed in the routine of healthcare institutions, and they are fully responsible for them.

2.7 CATEGORIES OF EDUCATIONAL NEEDS FOR NURSES

Nursing's role as an educator is extremely important, so it can't do without the opportunity to guide and instruct the client on what medication they are taking, why they are taking it, what the expected effects are and those that need to be warned about, informing them of possible allergies, acting as partners in this process and being able to prevent drug interactions.

It is possible to observe that these professionals do not supervise their team during the preparation and administration of medicines due to the high demand for services. It is up to the nurse to plan nursing actions, either with ideas, by providing adequate and safe material resources, by training the nursing team or by promoting adequate environmental and working conditions for the performance of their activities.

The education of the nursing team is extremely important for the prevention of medication errors. Therefore, prevention is directly related to education and knowledge, identifying and understanding the educational needs of nurses.

There are eight categories where nurses have the greatest need for knowledge and practice. These are

2.7.1 Mechanisms of action of medicines

It is worth noting that the terms action, effect and response are used synonymously and refer to the result of a drug's interaction with a biological entity in the body (BRODY, et. al. 1997).

It is therefore of fundamental importance for nurses to be aware of this category in order to promote educational actions. Currently, the administration of medicines requires knowledge of the mechanisms of action, responses relating to absorption, duration of the effect, metabolism and its relationship with half-life, bioavailability, elimination routes, the action of the drug in transplant clients and the absorption of the medicine through different routes.

It is one of the most outstanding, bringing together answers relating to absorption and duration of effect. In almost all cases, drugs must cross plasma membranes to reach their site of action. The ease with which a compound crosses membranes is the key to assessing the rates and extent of absorption and distribution of the drug in the body (BRODY, et. al. 1997).

Therefore, it is necessary to study this aspect of pharmacology and through this study nurses will be able to administer medicines more safely, minimizing the occurrence of medication errors and complications in clients arising from the administration of medicines.

2.7.2 Preparation and administration of medicines

Specifically with regard to dilution, it is known that different drugs require different volumes of diluent and that extreme cases of advanced age, impaired renal function, changes in blood pressure and hydroelectrolytic restriction should be observed. In these cases, a reduction in the recommended dilution volume should be considered (FAKIH, 2000).

This assessment facilitates the process of recovering customers, as it does not allow organs or systems to be further overloaded.

Another extremely important assessment for the administration of medicines is checking their expiry date. This is a relatively simple act that can prevent a medication error. With regard to the route of choice and the temperature at which the medicine should be administered, it is necessary to read the medical prescription and the package leaflet of the medicine in question very carefully.

Through the answers regarding dilution, shelf life, temperature, timing, infusion time and safety in the dosage of medicines.

There are also delays in administering the medication, as it is impossible to administer the medication on time due to the high demand from clients. However, in order to minimize this problem, it is necessary to prevent standardized schedules from being set for the same time, thus overloading the preparation and administration of medicines.

Obtaining information and knowledge about the drug administration process

It addresses the following aspects: information on pathologies, indications and contraindications, greater knowledge about drugs, equal relationship between trade name and scientific name, up-to-date description, pharmacology, indications, updating and active ingredients.

However, there was a lack of knowledge among nursing professionals regarding the medication to be administered. This is extremely contrary to what is recommended by scholars in the field of drug administration, since knowledge of the drug being administered is fundamental for the safe administration of drugs.

With regard to up-to-date information on knowledge and practices for administering medicines, technical knowledge in any field has become obsolete over the years. This implies a growing invasion of new technologies in everyday life, a fact that causes changes in the quantity, quality and speed of the exchange of information with which we live on a daily basis, in other words, requiring constant updating of these professionals (SHAPIRO; HUGHES,1996).

2.7.3 Prescription scheduling

Nurses play an important role in preventing medication errors during the scheduling of medical prescriptions. To carry out this task, nurses need to know the characteristics of the therapy and the client. When prescribing drugs administered orally, drug-food or drug-drug interactions must be prevented, especially in clients receiving nutritional therapy via gastric tubes.

With regard to intravenous therapy, it is the nurse's job to prevent possible incompatibilities that occur during the associated administration of drugs.

The nurse must be attentive to the schedule, distributing the medications so that they are not administered concomitantly, avoiding repeating the times of some medications such as: antibiotics, painkillers, antihypertensives, among others. In this respect, some precautions should be taken, for example, if the client is taking two antibiotics, distribute them over a 24-hour period, so that they have a satisfactory therapeutic result, as with the other medications. Another observation is not to put diuretic medications in at night, so as not to disturb the client's sleep and rest.

2.7.4 Drug interactions

It is important to note that the term *drug interactions* refers to an alteration in the magnitude or duration of the pharmacological response to a drug, due to the presence of another drug. It is essential that the nursing team, during drug therapy, observes and assesses the client for possible drug interactions and pharmacological incompatibilities, minimizing risks to the client (CARVALHO, 2000). The medication routine occupies a strategic position in precipitating these interactions.

2.7.5 Stability of medicines

It is important to check the drug manufacturer's specifications for the need for special care, as well as refrigeration, because for the same active ingredient, produced by different manufacturers, there may be variations in its stability after dilution and the shelf life of the drugs after preparation.

Photosensitivity related to the packaging of the drugs, which come in special packaging and the instructions for handling these drugs must be strictly followed.

2.7.6 Side effects of medicines

It is reported that drugs also activate the immune system in an undesirable way, causing allergic manifestations (BARBUTO, et. al. 1995). These reactions take the form of skin rashes, edema, anaphylactic reactions and fever. Nurses must be alert to these signs. They are the professionals responsible for informing the medical team, who will probably stop or replace the medication. This attitude is also possible and recommended when adverse reactions, side effects and allergic processes are observed.

Nurses who seek safe drug administration and are aware of side effects can act to minimize them as much as possible.

It should be emphasized that, in all matters relating to specific medicines, it is recommended to seek knowledge, i.e. to obtain information about each medicine. Only through in-depth study will it be possible to acquire a solid knowledge base, which will certainly represent an important achievement for nurses and their clients.

2.7.7 Other aspects of drug administration

The issue of iatrogenesis stands out, as following medication errors, the consequences for clients have been damage to the central nervous system, hypersensitivity reactions, amputation of limbs, decreased visual and hearing acuity, increased pain and may lead to the client's death (WOLF, et. al. 1996).

With regard to the routes of drug administration, it is known that this item depends on the characteristics of the effect expected by the team, and is subject to the routes of administration and the drug prescription.

2.8 PRACTICAL MEASURES FOR THE NURSING TEAM

Every day in nursing practice, despite the existence of institutionalized routines in relation to medications, it is possible and necessary to intervene in the way care is carried out, in order to prevent drug interactions and ensure a practice that is contextualized in science.

There are situations and activities related to the nursing team that need to be rethought and perhaps renewed. Examples of these situations are the planning of drug administration times in the medical prescription and the intervals between drugs, and practical measures should be adopted to help prevent adverse reactions resulting from interactions.

2.8.1 In parenteral infusions

- Avoid administering several drugs intravenously at the same time. Due to the greater possibility of drug interactions, potentiation or ineffectiveness of the drugs may occur;
- Avoid mixing medicines in the same solution or container, as this can alter their active ingredient;
- Avoid administering drugs that have the same toxic effects at the same time;
- Use different infusion routes when combining drugs of unknown or doubtful compatibility;
- Observe visible changes when reconstituting and diluting medicines (turbidity, precipitation, color change);
- Rinse infusion devices with neutral solutions, if available

the need to administer several drugs through the same vascular access route;

- Draw up a guide to drug incompatibilities with the agents most commonly used in the service and keep it in an easily accessible place;
- Consult your pharmacist if you have any doubts about unwanted effects or the compatibility of medicines.

2.8.2 When administering drugs enterally

- Avoid administering several drugs at the same time by enteral route;
- Avoid simultaneous administration of several tablets (oral or enteral tube);
- Observe an interval of approximately 2 hours when administering the medication;
- Always use the same vehicle (milk, fruit juice, water) when administering drugs that change their bioavailability;
- Avoid associating groups of "target drugs" and "precipitators" at the same times of administration.

2.9 LEGAL IMPLICATIONS FOR NURSING

Codes represent a collection of laws or regulations that govern human relations, assuring people of their rights, but also listing their duties. In this way, we can observe the codes that regulate the relationships between nurses and their clients/patients, in the convergent aspects relating to care practices in the medication process.

Article 12 of the Code of Ethics for Nursing Professionals states: "*Ensure that the person, family and community receive nursing care that is free from harm resulting from malpractice, negligence or recklessness*". This concept is in line with the Brazilian Civil Code, article 186, which states: "*Whoever, through voluntary action or omission, negligence or recklessness, violates a right and causes damage to another, even if exclusively moral, commits an unlawful act".* These aspects are reinforced by the Consumer Defense Code, which in article 6, chapter and item I, states: "*The basic rights of the consumer are: I - the protection of life, health and safety against the risks caused by practices in the supply of products and services considered dangerous or harmful".*

Despite the complexity of administering medication in nursing practice, this activity is most often carried out by mid-level professionals, nursing assistants and technicians, under the supervision and guidance of nurses. The act of delegating does not negate the responsibility that nurses have in meeting the care and health needs of the client as an individual, their family and significant others, even if they are carried out by their team. The nurse who is part of the hospital's staff is the natural or legal person who maintains this healthcare company, and they are respectively the agent and the principal.

Someone providing services under the orders of another or in obvious functional dependence (technical or administrative) is enough to characterize the relationship of preposition. The consequence of this is that both parties are jointly and severally liable for damages caused to the client. Therefore, nurses are also jointly and severally liable for damages caused if any of their subordinates, i.e. their employees, culpably harm a client.

In this sense, article 18 of the Code of Ethics for Nursing Professionals emphasizes that professionals must: "*Take responsibility for fault committed in their professional activities, regardless of whether it was practiced individually or as part of a team*". The Brazilian Civil Code, in article 951, provides for the obligation to compensate the victim when "... *in the case of compensation owed by anyone who, in the exercise of professional activity, through negligence, recklessness or malpractice, causes the death of the patient, aggravates his illness, causes him injury, or renders him unfit for work*". There is even the possibility that "... *if there is more than one perpetrator of the offense, all of them will be jointly and severally liable for the damages provided for in the consumer rules*".

Administering medication is one of the nursing team's greatest responsibilities. This means that this practice must be carried out in an appropriate and safe way for clients and that errors must therefore be prevented and avoided. Even though they have the legal support and curricular training to carry it out, it can be seen that professionals are often unprepared to do so, and that it can be carried out automatically and inattentively, disregarding the damage that an error in this process can cause.

In this context, even if the drug is safe in the intrinsic sense, it is the professional's duty to prevent adverse events and ensure safety in the use process. To ensure these aspects, it is essential for nurses to have a broad knowledge of the mode of action, adverse reactions and interactions of medicines. In this sense, article 30 of the Code of Ethics for Nursing Professionals prohibits nurses *from*: *"Administering medicines without knowing the action of the drug and without being sure of the possibility of risks".*

According to Law No. 7.498/86, which regulates the practice of nursing, in Article 11, Chapter II, nurses perform all nursing activities and are responsible for *prescribing medicines established in public health programs and in routines approved by the health institution.* Since the National Health Surveillance Agency (ANVISA) recognizes this attribution, as well as art. 4 of RDC No. 20/2011, it is clear that prescribing medication is the attribution of any or all legally qualified professionals, and is therefore not exclusively a medical act. This ANVISA resolution established what federal legislation had already provided for, that nurses should prescribe medicines that are part of the institution's programs or routine.

The managers of each dispensing unit cannot refuse to supply the medication prescribed by the nurse, as long as it is linked to the institution that has a program, public health protocols or routines approved by the health institution. In addition to administering drugs, nurses in some health institutions may prescribe some of these drugs. The need for nurses to know about medicines is therefore increasing in line with their duties.

Another ANVISA resolution, RDC No. 102/2000, in article 13, states: *"Any advertising, publicity or promotion of prescription medicines is restricted to the means of directed communication, aimed exclusively at health professionals, qualified to prescribe or dispense such products and must include"* and, in item I, indicates the information to which they refer, such as dosage, drug interactions, adverse reactions, among others.

It should be noted that the content of the current legislation, regarding the duties and responsibilities of nursing professionals in the provision of care; "*The nurse is responsible for administering medicines, prescribing nursing care in hospital, outpatient and home settings; The patient, their family or legal guardian must be advised of the therapy that will be implemented, objectives, risks, routes of administration and possible complications that may arise; It is the nurse's responsibility to ensure that all occurrences and data relating to the patient and their treatment are recorded correctly, guaranteeing the availability of the information needed to evaluate the patient, make the treatment effective and track adverse events",* among others.

3. METHODOLOGY

3.7 TYPE OF STUDY

In this study we opted for a descriptive qualitative approach, which according to Chizzotti (2001) refers to qualitative research as that based on data extracted from interpersonal interactions, co-participation in the situations of the informants, analyzed based on the meaning they give to their actions. The researcher participates, understands and interprets. According to Minayo (2007, p.57):

> The qualitative method is applied to the study of history, relationships, representations, beliefs, perceptions and opinions, products of the interpretations that humans make about how they live, build their artifacts and themselves, feel and think.

Regarding field research, Lakatos and Marconi (2007, p.188) explain that:

> Field research is research used with the aim of obtaining information and/or knowledge about a problem to which an answer is sought, or a hypothesis that is to be proven, or to discover new phenomena or the relationships between them.

3.8 RESEARCH SCENARIO

The study was carried out in a private hospital located in the metropolitan region of Belém. The hospital offers medium and high complexity care. Its physical structure consists of: Laboratory; X-rays; Ultrasound; Urgent and Emergency Care; Clinical and Surgical Hospitalization; Adult and Pediatric Intensive Care Units (ICU). It has 56 active beds distributed among these services and 23 nurses on staff. The hospital was chosen after the internship was carried out on its premises, due to its demand and the flow of medicines administered.

3.9 RESEARCH SUBJECTS

The subjects of the survey were twenty-three (23) nurses from the hospital. The sample consisted of twenty (20) nurses who answered the questionnaire. The inclusion criteria were nurses who were employees and agreed to take part in the research, and the exclusion criteria were not being an employee nurse and not agreeing to take part in the research. We chose to use the letter E, followed by a numerical order from 1 to 20 according to the order in which the data was collected.

3.10 ETHICAL CONDUCT OF RESEARCH

This research was guided by Resolution 196/96 of the National Health Council, which regulates research on human beings. It was approved by the Ethics Committee - No. 432427/11 (ANNEX A).

The participants were explained the need to sign the Free and Informed Consent Form (Appendix A), which contains information about the research: the subject, objectives, method, risks and benefits; guaranteeing anonymity and confidentiality with regard to identification and also ensuring the free right to participate or not in the research, leaving it without any loss whatsoever.

3.11 DATA COLLECTION

After signing the informed consent form, data collection began, using an interview script that was recorded with the subjects' authorization. Minayo (1998, p.108) explains that:

> The interview is a privileged instrument for collecting data, because the word is an essential object in communication, and is capable of revealing the structural conditions, systems, values, norms and symbols of a specific culture. In addition, the interview has the capacity to capture "non-verbalized" reactions, such as gestures, silence, an expression. All worthy of consideration.

The profile of the subjects, knowledge and practice of drug interaction (APPENDIX B), selected the following variables for the study: drug action, drug reaction, side effects and drug interaction.

3.12 DATA ANALYSIS

The material collected was transcribed and analyzed using the content analysis method, as it is the method that allows us to operationalize the treatment of data and, consequently, to systematize, analyze and interpret it in a qualitative way.

According to Bardin (1977, p.35), content analysis can be defined as:

> A set of communication analysis techniques aimed at obtaining, through systematic and objective procedures for describing the content of messages, indicators (quantitative or not) that allow the interference of knowledge related to the conditions of production/reception of these messages.

The analysis was carried out by questioning the nurses and their responses on the topic "Drug Interaction: Knowledge and Practice of Nurses". An analysis was made of the results obtained through the interviews with the nurses in the study, as well as a reflection on the topic, considering the relevant points to encourage other researchers on the subject.

3.13 ANALYSIS OF THE RISKS AND BENEFITS OF THE RESEARCH

The research offered minimal risk, as it was only a risk inherent in carrying out the research project, since in accordance with Law 196/96° their names were preserved.

The research did not unduly expose or harm those involved in any way. The research subjects did not have their data disclosed, the professional's information was kept confidential, and at the end of the research, the data collection form was filed and will be dispensed with after a period of five years, until which time it will be kept by CLAYSE JENNIFER ALVES DE SOUZA, a student on the Nursing Degree Course at the University of Amazonia.

We can cite the following benefits: an increase in scientific production by nurses on the subject in question; providing nurses with specific knowledge in order to better plan nursing care; and arousing the interest of the academic community and existing professionals in paying better attention to the discipline of Pharmacology; so that there is greater knowledge and better training of nurses on drug interactions, thus improving the quality of care and minimizing possible risks to the client, even reducing their time in hospital and the cost of treatment for the health institution.

4. Analysis AND DISCUSSION OF RESULTS

This chapter presents the analysis of the data obtained in the research, carried out by applying the questionnaires to the subjects involved in the process.

4.7 SOCIO-DEMOGRAPHIC PROFILE

Twenty nurses (ET = 20) contributed to the study. The socio-demographic profile of these subjects was drawn up as follows:

Table 1 - Distribution of interviewees according to age group. Belém-PA, 2011.

Age	Total	%
25 to 30 years	4	20
31 to 36 years old	9	45
37 to 42 years old	5	25
43 to 48 years old	2	10
Total	**20**	**100**

Source: Souza, C. J. A. 2011.

Of the twenty people interviewed, 20% were aged between 25 and 30, 45% were aged between 31 and 36, 25% were aged between 37 and 42 and 10% were aged between 43 and 48, i.e. the majority of professionals were young.

Table 2 - Distribution of interviewees according to length of professional training. Belém-

PA, 2011.

Time since graduation	Total	%
0 to 5 years	5	25
6 to 11 years	8	40
12 to 17 years	5	25
18 to 23 years old	2	10
Total	**20**	**100**

Source: Souza, C. J. A. 2011.

Of the twenty nurses interviewed, 25% have been trained for between 0 and 05 years, 40% have been trained for between 6 and 11 years, 25% have been trained for between 12 and 17 years and 10% have been trained for between 18 and 23 years. The majority have been trained for a significant period of time.

Table 3 - Distribution of interviewees according to length of service in the institution. Belém-PA, 2011.

Length of Service	Total	%
0 to 2 years	11	55
3 to 5 years	5	25
6 to 8 years	4	20
Total	**20**	**100**

Source: Souza, C. J. A. 2011.

Of the twenty nurses interviewed, 55% have between 0 and 2 years' service, 25% have between 3 and 5 years' service and 20% have between 6 and 8 years' service. Most of them, 55%, have only been working in this health institution for a short time.

4.8 Thematic questions

Table 1 - Drug action, drug reaction and drug side effects.

Answers	Action of Medicines	Drug reactions	Side Effects of Medicines
Yes	16	15	4

No	0	3	14
In part	4	2	2

Source: Souza, C. J. A. 2011.

However, when studying nursing professionals with regard to their lack of knowledge, it was found that the majority have little knowledge of the medication to be administered (CARVALHO, 2000). nurses must know the indications and contraindications, the trade name and scientific name, and especially the active ingredient.

As the years go by, nurses' knowledge becomes outdated and they become professionals without a scientific basis. In order for this not to happen, these professionals have to be constantly updated to provide their clients with quality care with the minimum of possibilities and occurrences of harm to the client.

The greater the nurse's knowledge of the drugs they administer, the greater their ability to develop drug administration (OPTIZ, 2002).

Nurses are higher education professionals whose curriculum includes pharmacology, and they are the only professionals in the nursing team who should have sufficient knowledge to conduct this practice safely (SILVA, et al. 2007).

Most of the time, undergraduates lack interest in the subject of pharmacology, and during internships, drug therapy becomes a major source of fear, anxiety and insecurity. These feelings emerge when students are faced with such immense responsibility for dealing with lives, and this is reflected after they become professionals. Here's the question: Are undergraduate nursing courses preparing students to carry out drug therapy? Is the pharmacology taught in a single semester enough?

During the survey, the nurses reported that the pharmacology they learned during the nursing course at university was incipient, that in one semester, we can't learn everything that is required of us as professionals, having to learn it on a daily basis, in the practical routines of nursing.

The reaction of medicines in our bodies is based on how they work, as well as their absorption, distribution, metabolization or excretion. In all matters relating to specific medicines, it is advisable to search for knowledge, i.e. to obtain information about each medicine. Only through in-depth study will it be possible to acquire a solid basis, which will certainly represent a great achievement for nurses and their clients (TELLES; CASSIANI, 2004).

Side effects are responses resulting from the interaction which can lead to an increase in the therapeutic effect, a decrease in efficacy, the appearance of adverse reactions which can be severe or minor, or even cause no change in the desired effect of the drug.

The client can be alerted to any signs and symptoms that may indicate an adverse effect, as many of these clients use concomitant medications that interact with each other without showing any evidence of an adverse effect.

According to ANVISA's RDC No. 47/O9, which states that all medicines must have a package leaflet, Art. 1 approves the Technical Regulation that establishes the minimum requirements for the preparation, harmonization, updating, publication and availability of package leaflets for medicines for patients and health professionals.

Art. 2 This Regulation aims to improve the form and content of the package leaflets of all registered and notified medicines marketed in Brazil, in order to guarantee access to safe and adequate information for the rational use of medicines.

Chart 2 - Nurses' knowledge of drug interactions.

Answers	**Nurses' Knowledge of Drug Interactions**
They know	5
Do You Have Any Idea	6
Could not answer	9

Source: Souza, C. J. A. 2011.

Definition of the answers obtained:

*"Based on the antibiogram, which will be the line drug and monitor whether it continues or not (Unknown)". **(E3)***

*"What do you mean, drug interaction?" **(E4)***

*"The way a medication reacts with another drug." **(E6)***

*"The administration of several medicines in which one can potentiate the action of the other." **(E9)***

*"You can't administer drugs together to avoid unwanted effects." **(E11 / E12)***

According to the answers, we can see that the majority of interviewees are unaware of the subject, while some have heard of it or have some idea of it. The minority are aware of drug interactions and are attentive to them in their day-to-day nursing work. According to Hoefler (2008), drug interactions are clinical events in which the effects of a drug are altered by the presence of another drug, food, drink or some environmental chemical agent.

When two drugs are administered concomitantly to a patient, they can act independently or interact with each other, with an increase or decrease in the therapeutic or toxic effect of one or the other.

The conclusion of a drug interaction can be dangerous when it promotes an increase in the toxicity of a drug.

We can see that the answers to the first questions on the thematic axis don't match up with the answers to the fourth question, where most of the interviewees answered "YES" to the conviction that they know the medicines they administer and how they react in the body. As a result, we can see that nurses are administering medicines according to what they have learned over their professional experience, doing so automatically with the minimum possible knowledge, in a worrying way that could cause eminent risk for the client and for themselves in terms of legal implications.

Chart 3 - Answers obtained on the scheduling of medication.

Answers	**Take Medicines at the Same Times**
Yes	6
No	14

Source: Souza, C. J. A. 2011.

Definition of the answers obtained:

*"No, according to the routine of each hospital. Care with antibiotics and psychotropic drugs." **(E3)***

*"No, never! We take a 5-minute break when we have two drugs to administer at the same time. " **(E4)***

*"No, they try to make it comfortable for the client during the hours, they try to organize the hours so that they don't interact." **(E17)***

*"Yes (I didn't know what scheduling meant)." **(E2)***

*"Yes, it depends on the medicine." **(E6)***

*"Yes, as long as there is no harm to the patient. " **(E9)***

It is the job of nurses to schedule administration times based on the prescription, the policy of their institution and the relevant characteristics of the medication itself (CABRAL, 2002).

We can see that the majority of those interviewed answered that they don't take their medication at the same times, but only one had any idea why they didn't do so. Incompatibility between active ingredients must be taken into account when scheduling prescribed medicines (FAKIH, 2002).

Of those who answered "YES", one didn't know what it meant to make an appointment, while others gave vague answers as to why they could.

Table 4 - Responses obtained on the supervision of medication administration.

Answers	**Supervising the administration of medicines**
Yes	8
No	10
Whenever possible	2

Source: Souza, C. J. A. 2011.

Definition of the answers obtained:

"It's not possible, due to the demand for services." ***(E18)***

"Not always because of the amount of work." ***(E16)***

The legislation for the professional practice of nursing, through Decree Law No. 94.406/87 in its article 8, which provides for the exclusive duties of nurses, determines in the COREN lines.

4.9 organizing and directing nursing services and their technical and auxiliary activities in companies providing these services.

4.10 planning, organizing, coordinating, executing and evaluating nursing care services.

In article 11, the decree explains the duties of the auxiliary, in item III and especially in line "a", it legalizes the action of administering drugs orally and parenterally, and together with article 13, it determines that this activity can only be carried out under the supervision, guidance and direction of the nurse (COREN-SP, 1996).

By analyzing the content of these articles, we understand that, although some functions of caring for human beings are delegated to the nursing team, it is the nurse's responsibility to be involved in all the actions carried out by any component of his or her subordination. The act of delegating does not negate the nurse's responsibility for nursing care and caring for the client's health, as they are responsible for the care provided by their team.

4.10.1 Criteria for Supervision

Another point highlighted was the criteria used to supervise:

"They didn't answer. " ***(E1 / E3 / E12 / E17 / E20)***

"Selection of patients who require greater care, such as: extremes of age or critically ill patients. " ***(E9)***

"The right five in nursing: the right route, the right medication, the right dose, the right patient, the right time, and today there are nine right ones." ***(E7/E8)***

"The degree of importance of the medication, for example, if it's something I don't know or if it's new on the market." ***(E13)***

"Observes the preparation of the medication and its administration when he is around. " ***(E16)***

"Check the medical records to see if they have been done. " ***(E18)***

We can see that there were many different answers and that most of them had no supervision criteria. According to Elliott (2010), many care tasks involve a degree of risk and the administration of medication undoubtedly carries a great deal of risk, so it is necessary to continuously evaluate all stages of drug therapy, which should be carried out primarily by nursing staff.

In the process of administering medication, nurses used to use the 5 right things (patient, drug, route, dose, right time) as an evaluation strategy. Recently, this has been increased to 7 right things, adding documentation and the action of the drug administered, and the most innovative study complements this strategy with 9 right things, including the form and the right answer (ELLIOTT, 2010). Evaluation strategies do not prevent errors from occurring, but they do minimize their possibilities by highlighting the risks and allowing action to be taken on them.

5. FINAL CONSIDERATIONS

- There is a need to wake up to the importance of drug administration, which brings with it drug interactions. Due to nurses' lack of knowledge, these go unnoticed in nursing routines, and when they occur, they result in harm to the client and the professional, who ends up facing ethical questions about this practice. Nurses must be able to describe and identify interactions and suggest appropriate interventions, as well as individualizing recommendations based on a client's specific parameters.
- Health services such as hospitals, clinics and home care companies must be committed to providing professionals with an information system that allows them to practice safely, and should focus on medication strategies, as this is the most common form of intervention in health care and the most common cause of adverse events, many of which are avoidable.
- Any substance ingested by the individual without the intention of promoting a therapeutic effect (such as food, alcohol or tobacco) could lead to drug interactions with any medication the individual is using, causing alterations in the therapeutic efficacy and toxicity

of these substances.

- Research reveals the importance of training and improving nurses' knowledge of drug administration content and its interactions, and nothing could be more appropriate than examining nurses' training: there is a need to deepen their undergraduate knowledge of pharmacology content and integrate it into their practice.

- The institution should propose training aimed at meeting professional needs through studies and evidence, in order to update knowledge about the difficulties identified in the knowledge and practice of drug interactions.

BIBLIOGRAPHICAL REFERENCES

ASPERHEIM. M. K. **Farmacologia para Enfermagem**. 7ª ed Rio de Janeiro: Guanabara Koogan,1992.

BARBUTO, J.A.M.; HERSH, E.M.; SALMON, S.E. **Immunopharmacology.** In Katzung BG, Silva P. Farmacologia bàsica & clinica. Rio de Janeiro (RJ): Guanabara Koogan; 1995. p. 656-71.

BARDIN, L. **Content Analysis.** Lisbon, Ediçôes 70, p.35, 1977.

BOECHAT, NS. **Drug interaction in the elderly.** *J* Bras Med., v. 60, n.4, p.75-83, 1991.

BRAZIL. LAW No. 10.406, of January 10, 2002. **Establishes the Brazilian Civil Code.**

BRAZIL. LAW No. 8078, of September 11, 1990. **Provides for consumer protection and other measures.**

BRODY TM, Larner J, Minneman KP, Neu HC. **Human pharmacology: from molecular to clinical**. 2nd edition. Rio de Janeiro (RJ): Guanabara Koogan; 1997.

CAMPOS, E.R.C.; BARDINA, N.B.; VEJA, M.A. **Interacciones medicamentosas: errores En La Medicacion.** Rev Cubana Farm, v.24, n.2, p.281-7, 1990.

CARVALHO VT. **Errors in the administration of medication: an analysis of reports by nursing professionals.** [Dissertation]. Ribeirao Preto (SP): Ribeirao Preto Nursing School/USP; 2000.

CABRAL, I. E. **Administraçâo de medicamentos.** Rio de Janeiro: Reichmann & Affonso Editores, 2002.

REGIONAL NURSING COUNCIL-COREN (BR-SP). **Main legislation for the practice of nursing.** Sâo Paulo: COREN; 1996.

FEDERAL NURSING COUNCIL. **COFEN Resolution No. 311/2007. Approves the**

Reformulation of the Code of Ethics for Nursing Professionals. [cited in: 01 Apr 2008].

CORBETT, C. E. **The pharmacological bases for therapeutics**. 6ª edition, Guanabara Koogan, 1982.

COSTA, P.D. The **need to know about drug interactions.** Arq. Bras. Med., v. 58, n.3, p.157-9, 1984.

CHIZZOTTI, A. **Pesquisa em Ciências Humanas e Sociais.** 5.ed. São Paulo: Cortez, 2001.

EISENBERG, S. **Intravenous drug compatibility: a challenge for the oncology nurse**. Oncol Nurs Forum,v 24, n.5, p.85969, 1997.

ELLIOTT, M; LIU,Y. **The nine rights of medication administration: an overview.** British Journal of Nursing, Vol 19, 2010.

FAKIH F. T. **Manual of dilution and administration of injectable drugs.**

Rio de Janeiro (RJ): Reichman & Afonso; 2000.

FAKIH, F. T. **Manual of dilution and administration of injectable medicines**.

São Paulo: Reichmann & Affonso Editores, 2002.

FONSECA, A.L. **Interações medicamentosas.** Rio de Janeiro, EPUC, 1994.

GRAHAME-SMITH, D.G.; ARONSON, J.K. **Oxford textbook of clinical pharmacology and drug therapy.** Oxford, Oxford University Press, 1988. Chap 10, p.158-71: Drug interactions.

HARADA, M.J.C.S.; PEDREIRA, M.L.G.; PETERLINI, M.A.S.; PEREIRA, S.R. **O erro humano e a segurança do paciente**. 2° edição. Atheneu Publishing House, 2007.

HOEFLER, R. **Drug interactions**. National Therapeutic Formulary. Secretariat of Science, Technology and Strategic Supplies/MS - FTN. Ministry of Health. Brasilia-DF, 2008.

HUSSAR, D.A **Drug Interactions**. In: GENNARO, A.R. Remington: the science and practice of pharmacy. 20 ed., Baltimore: Lippincott Williams & Wilkins, 2000. p.1746-61

LAKATOS, E. M.; MARCONI, M. A. **Fundamentos de Metodologia Cientifica** 6ª ed. São Paulo: Atlas, 2007.

MADUREIRA, C.R.; VEIGA K.; SANT'ANA A.F.M. **Management of technology in intensive care unit.** Rev. Latino Enf. 2000.

MENGARDO, S.; OGUISSO, T. **Drug interactions and nursing.** Rev Paul Hosp, n.4/5/6, p.75-80, 1986.

MIASSO, A. I.; CASSIANI, S. H. DE B. **Errors in the administration of medication: dissemination of knowledge and identification of the patient as relevant aspects.** Rev.Esc.Enf.USP, v. 34, n. 1, p. 16-25, mar. 2000.

MINAYO, M. C. S. **O desafio do conhecimento: pesquisa qualitativa em saù.** Sâo Paulo:Hucitec, p.57, 2007.

MINAYO, M. C. S. **O desafio do conhecimento: Pesquisa qualitativa em saù.** 5 ed. Sâo Paulo- Rio de Janeiro: Hucitec- Abrasco, p. 108, 1998.

NIES, A.S.; SPIELBERG, S.E. Principles of Therapeutics. In: GOODMAN;

GILMAN'S. **The Pharmacological Basis of Therapeutcs.** 9th New York, Mc Graw- Hill, 1996.Chap.3, p.43-62.

OGA, S.; BASILE, A.C. **Medicines and their interactions**. Sâo Paulo, Atheneu, 1994.

OPTIZ, S.P. **Understanding the meaning of medication administration for undergraduate nursing students.** [Dissertation]. Ribeirâo Preto (SP): Ribeirâo Preto Nursing School/USP; 2002.

POTTER, P. A.; PERRY, A. G. **Fundamentals of Nursing**. Rio de Janeiro: Guanabara Koogan, 2001.

SHAPIRO, J.; HUGHES, S. **Information technology as a liberal art.** Educ. Rev. 1996.

SECOLI, SR. **Drug interactions: foundations for clinical nursing practice**. Rev. Esc. Enf. USP**,** v.35, n. 1, p. 28-34, mar. 2001.

SILVA A.E.B. **Análisis do sistema de** medicaçâo **de um hospital universitàrio do estado de Goiàs**. [Dissertation]. Ribeirao Preto (SP): Ribeirao Preto Nursing School/USP; 2003.

SILVA, D.O.; GROU, C.R.; MIASSO, A.I.; CASSIANI, S.H.B. **Preparation and administration of medication: analysis of questions and information from the nursing team.** Rev. Latino-am de Enfermagem 2007 September-October.

TATRO, D.S. **Drug Interaction Facts 1999**. St.Louis: Facts and Comparisons, 1999.

TELLES P.C.P.Filho; CASSIANI S.H.B. **Administraçâo de medicamentos: aquisiçâo de conhecimento e habilidades requeridas por um grupo de enfermeiros.** Rev. Latino-am Enfermagem 2004 May-June.

THOMPSON, J.H. Drug interactions. In: BEVAN, J.A. **Fundamentos de farmacologia.** Sao Paulo, Harper and Row do Brasil, 1979. Chap.4, p.24-9.

WOLF, Z.R.; MCGOLDRIK, T.B.; FLYNN, E.R.; WARNICK, F. **Factors associated with a perceived harmful outcome from medication errors: a pilot study.** J Contin Educ Nurs, 1996.

CHAPTER III - THE STUDY OF THE FATHER'S PSYCHOEMOTIONAL ASPECTS DURING THE PUERPERAL GRAPHIC CYCLE

HISIS DA COSTA SOUSA

JEAN JORGE DA SILVA FERREIRA MARIA LUCIANA OLIMPIO DA SILVA

MARIA TITA PORTAL SACARMENTO

SUMMARY

Reflections on the father's active participation in the puerperal pregnancy cycle, his role in the family context, and the insertion of the baby in the formation of a new family, led us to discuss the meaning of the father figure and what changes might be occurring in the face of the diversity of family arrangements and the many socio-cultural contexts that are mixed together. The aim of this research is to analyze the father's participation, experience and emotions during pregnancy and the birth of his child, to explain the father's participation during pregnancy and birth, to report on the father's psycho-emotional aspects during the birth of his child and to evaluate the father's emotional involvement at the time of the birth. This is a descriptive qualitative case study. The fathers interviewed described how, when they found out they were going to be fathers, they were overcome with emotion. They took an active part in all the stages of pregnancy and childbirth, and reported that all their fears and anxieties were calmed when they held their child in their arms. It is hoped that this research will contribute to the teaching and research perspectives of health professionals and parents who seek out this topic, helping to improve care in health practices. In conclusion, this research has enabled us to study issues peculiar to men in the context of being a father and that their participation in all stages of pregnancy and birth is fundamental to establishing an early bond between father and child, as well as providing comfort and security for their partner and the baby at the time of delivery. **Keywords:** Obstetric Nursing; Humanized Childbirth; Companion.

1 INTRODUCTION

The event of a pregnancy presents factors far beyond biological transformations in the female body, because associated with these transformations there is a mixture of sensations or feelings that weave this moment both physically and emotionally for the couple and everyone around them at this unique moment in a couple's life (BRANDÂO, 2009).

During the practical classes in Women's Health, especially with regard to prenatal care, the absence of the father at this very important moment in pregnancy was what most caught our attention. The father's participation in the woman's labor had positive consequences for the birth and for building the bond between the father and the newborn.

According to Oliveira (2007), fathers at the time of childbirth allow both themselves and their wives to experience the birth of their child together, an important moment in their married life. Fathers, both those who are experiencing this for the first time and those who have already taken part, have certainly remembered that the birth of a child is a unique moment in their lives. Regardless of this, the experience of accompanying the birth should be so rewarding that they should understand that it is their duty to accompany the woman during the birth process, and that this participation provides security and support for the parturient woman, avoiding possible complications.

According to da Silva Tarnowskil; Próspero; Elsen (2005) men, raised from a young age to be macho, tough, providers and protectors, are suddenly asked to be sensitive, collaborative and even "maternal" towards their pregnant wives and babies. Raised to compete in the jungle of the job market, he is now asked to wash bottles and change diapers. Raised to provide, he is now expected to take turns with his wife in caring for the baby, while she goes out, works and earns her own money. The woman, brought up from an early age to be soft, sensitive, understanding and gentle, is suddenly expected to be indifferent, competitive, aggressive in the job market and to progress professionally. Until she has a baby, because then she is expected to drop everything and 'mother' her baby, at least for a while, while the children are so small and need their mother so much.

Traditionally, the role of the father was seen only as the breadwinner of the family, the one who worked to support the family, with the role of the woman as the main caretaker of the home, the children and the husband. This model, now in disuse, is due to the inversion of the role of women in society, who are entering the job market, seeking a more active position in all fields of work, balancing domestic activities and a professional career, but these rights have not been granted to them so easily, However, these rights were not granted to them so easily, but they became more visible from the 1960s onwards, when Labra (1989) said that the development of contraceptive methods and the dissemination of their use were partly responsible for the change in women's lives and social roles, giving them greater access to the job market and sexual freedom, which they were still unaware of (LEITE *et al*, 2009).

In Brazil, in 1975, actions were formalized to provide assistance during pregnancy, childbirth and the puerperium, to encourage breastfeeding, as well as measures for spacing pregnancies, aimed at women between the ages of 15 and 49, who were considered to be part of the most vulnerable groups according to criteria based on the concept of risk. One of the aims of these actions was to prevent and treat controllable diseases, through technologies such as immunization, food supplementation and monitoring of less medically complex problems, such as parasites, anaemia, urinary infections and hypertension, also aiming, among other things, to reduce the number of maternal deaths (MATTAR; DINIZ, 2012).

Currently, a new vision of these rights is based on a context of humanization, which aims to cover all fields of law, whether for couples or individuals, One of the main ones is maternity leave of 120 days for women, and men in the same gestational context also have the opportunity to be covered by various other laws, ranging from accompanying women at all stages of the pregnancy cycle and especially at the time of childbirth, where it is necessary for hospital institutions to ensure compliance with Law No. 11. 108, enacted on April 7, 2005.108, enacted on April 7, 2005, which ensures the presence of a companion of the woman's choice during the birth process (BRASIL, 2014).

According to Brasil (2005), women can choose to have a companion with whom they have a bond to be by their side during labor, childbirth or the immediate postpartum period, so the man (husband) appears to be the best option to accompany them during childbirth, but regardless of whether or not he is the companion, he, the father, is legally entitled to 5 days of paternity leave, and there are also bills going through the national congress to make better use of this father during the postpartum period.

The need to research and discuss the importance of the father's presence at the birth of his child arose as there is a perception that the majority of this population is unaware of their rights to participate from prenatal care to childbirth. This study will also seek to provide scientific basis for better assistance in health practices.

3 OBJECTIVES

3.1 General Objective

- To analyze the father's participation, experience and emotions during pregnancy and the birth of his child.

3.2 Specific Objectives

- Explain the father's role during pregnancy and birth;
- Reporting on the psycho-emotional aspects of fathers during the birth of their children;
- Evaluating the father's emotional involvement at the time of birth.

4 THEORETICAL BASIS

4.1 Birth History

Childbirth is considered to be a watershed in a woman's life, full of meanings that are constructed and reconstructed based on the singularity and culture of the woman giving birth, which transforms her daily life. Historically, labor and childbirth took place in the home environment, "this process is an event in which the art of giving birth took place in the woman's home, which was usually accompanied by a midwife she trusted, in this scenario, the woman freely expressed her feelings and desires in a warm environment within the family (BRUGGEMANN, *et al*, 2005).

Traditionally, the act of childbirth involved handing over the parturient woman to a midwife, who acquired her techniques by delivering babies on her own or after learning from other midwives, and usually in an empirical way. Learning therefore takes place in practice, in a context of a lack of assistance for pregnant women, in which the midwife acts autonomously. For the most part, midwives are driven by a desire to serve, by a feeling of solidarity and this practice adds a good deal of experience to them, which in this context becomes relevant, centralizing the act of childbirth only in the parturient woman assisted by a midwife (NASCIMENTO *et al*, 2009).

However, for a long time, not only did midwifery pose real risks to the mother and the fetus, but so did doctors: in 1878, it was estimated that English women had a six-fold increase in their chances of dying when they were admitted to maternity wards in England. More accessible to working class women, the traditional midwife was involved in domestic chores, replacing or assisting the woman for a month or more after childbirth. The dispute over the hegemony of childbirth care was marked by two episodes involving midwives, with major repercussions for current Western models of childbirth care. "One of them, which took place in England, culminated in the incorporation of their work into the official health system: the passing of the Midwives Act of 1902." The other, in the United States of America, led to the transformation of the work of midwives into a practice outside the law, based on the strategy of holding them responsible for the high rates of maternal and perinatal mortality at the beginning of the 20th century, known as the *"midwife problem"* (OSAWA *et al*, 2006).

As in other parts of the world, in Brazil in 2005, with the creation of the Undergraduate Obstetrics Course at the University of São Paulo, the discussions around models for training non-medical professionals in childbirth care were focused on establishing their hegemony in the health field and disputing the midwife's clientele. For a long time, the surgeon's participation in childbirth was seen as something degrading, and the midwife's job was considered dishonorable and vile, because it dealt with female secretions and odors. The entry requirements for childbirth courses were lower than for other courses. As well as being treated as a less literate activity than medicine, it was the only course that required its candidates to have a certificate of "good manners" (OSAWA *et al*, 2006).

4.2 Humanizing Childbirth

Pregnancy is a new and intense event in a couple's life and is considered a unique experience. Childbirth is an explosion of feelings involving the family, especially the parents. It is a transitional phase, where feelings are mixed with anxiety and preparation for the birth of the baby, and new roles emerge. Each person can have multiple experiences and new sensations with the arrival of the new member, and it is necessary to work on their psycho-emotional reception so that they are ready for the changes, and that this special moment is pleasant and peaceful, contributing to a positive experience for both (PERDOMINI; BONILHA, 2011).

The question of the best way to give birth is an issue that has been discussed worldwide for a long time. Nowadays, there is a lot of talk about natural or normal childbirth, which translates into humanized childbirth, as well as the controversial caesarean section. Studies show that childbirth, regardless of the technique, should be decided by the woman giving birth, who is the person who will actually undergo the procedure (PETITO *et al*, 2015).

The institutionalization of childbirth took place shortly after the Second World War with the aim of minimizing the maternal and infant mortality rate. This model prioritized health professionals and institutional norms, automatically removing the parturient during labour and childbirth from her family. Because of this distancing, some private and especially public hospitals began to develop actions that referred to humanization, bringing with these actions more comfort to the parturient and her family, but hospital norms remained dominant (RIOS, 2009).

According to OLIVEIRA, *et al* 2002, it was in an attempt to recover the physiological nature of childbirth that the concept of humanized childbirth emerged, with the aim of promoting healthy childbirth and births and preventing maternal and perinatal morbidity and mortality. As a result, institutions and health workers have returned to the real concept of childbirth, where it is a normal physiological process, but where the emotional aspects are fundamental and must be respected (SÓNIA, 2009).

Humanized care gives women a strong sense of confidence and security during childbirth and when caring for their child. Many have a wonderful experience of self-transformation, feeling capable in their new social role. This experience stimulates awareness and interest in society, resulting in social empowerment. The World Health Organization proposes the humanization of childbirth care with the aim of promoting healthy labour and birth and the prevention of maternal and perinatal mortality, with careful interventions, avoiding excesses in the use of available technological resources. Childbirth is a remarkable experience for women and can leave positive or negative memories such as suffering, fear of becoming pregnant again and depression (PETITO *et al*, 2015).

Studies have shown the physical and psychological benefits that the humanized care model brings to women, changing the social concept of childbirth. Humanizing childbirth means putting the woman at the center and in control as the subject of her actions, participating intimately and actively in decisions about her own care. In this way, the team acts as a facilitator of the process (SILVA *et al*, 2009).

In 1998, the Ministry of Health began to implement a series of initiatives and incentives aimed at humanizing issues, with the aim of improving the quality of obstetric care, revaluing normal childbirth, reducing the rate of unnecessary caesarean sections, a model that has been growing over the last few decades, and strengthening the mother's relationship with her baby (BRASIL, 1999).

As a result of these changes, humanization was born within the SUS, leading the Ministry of Health to create the National Program for the Humanization of Hospital Care (PNHAH), where this program disseminates ideas and promotes humanization actions. In 2003, the Ministry of Health revised the program and launched the National Humanization Program (PNH), which extended its reach to the entire SUS network, making the National Humanization Policy act on the basis of clinical, ethical and political guidelines, which translate into certain working arrangements (SERRUYA *et al,* 2005).

"The obstetric service provider" must have adequate training and a variety of obstetric skills appropriate to the level of care and be able to carry out essential basic interventions and care for the newborn after birth. They should refer the mother or newborn to a more complex level of care if complications arise that require interventions beyond their competence (SERRUYA, 2004).

Parturient health care has been discussed with a view to making the process of giving birth a context for promoting the health of women and their newborns, as natural as possible and with the aim of inhibiting the excess of surgical deliveries. It is just one of the goals of this assistance, which should be consolidated if it is built with a focus on more humanized care. The health professionals who care for this population have been identified as important mediators in making this proposal a reality. The current protocols call for highly trained professionals, so developments in the search for knowledge in the obstetric field have become mandatory for these professionals, leading to a significant change in both professional training and care for this clientele, so that professionals need to be up to date on the changes and especially in practicing the laws that govern the care and rights of the patient (REIS; PATRICIO, 2006).

The beneficial nature of continuous support during childbirth has been proven with the insertion of a companion from the woman's social network, which contributes to an increase in spontaneous vaginal deliveries, a reduction in the need for intrapartum analgesia, dissatisfaction/negative perception of the birth experience, the duration of labor, caesarean sections, instrumental vaginal deliveries and newborns with low Apgar scores. Furthermore, paternal participation in the birth process contributes to improving the parturient's self-control and strengthening the family bond, as well as ensuring a wider range of support (FIGUEIREDO, 2011).

Article 198 of the Federal Constitution and Organic Law 8080, of September 19, 1990, regulate the Unified Health System and provide for the principle of the right to information about the health of users, extended to their families and companions, in a clear, objective, respectful and understandable manner, as well as the preservation of autonomy in the defense of their physical and moral integrity (BRASIL, 2007).

It is known that the quality of the support provided by the companion is almost always proportional to their ability to be more active in the birthing process, and it is clear that it is important to develop educational technologies aimed at instructing them, allowing them to expand their role of support and active participation in childbirth (FRUTUOSO, 2005).

Law 11.108/2005, or the Accompanying Person Law, guarantees the right of every pregnant woman to be accompanied during prepartum, childbirth and the postpartum period. Another right that parturient women have is respect for their autonomy. This is the right of every service user, and is indisputable in the health sector. Autonomy is the person's right to have their own opinions, make their own choices and act on the basis of personal values and beliefs, to communicate with family members, and to guarantee information about the care process that takes place inside the obstetric center (BRASIL, 2005).

Despite the legislation in force and the recognized importance of the companion during labor and delivery, some barriers hinder the consolidation of this practice, such as inadequate physical space, lack of acceptance by some professional categories and the failure of pregnant women to demand their rights, Another aggravating factor is the limited number of measures that promote the autonomy of the companion to participate in this period, and no training process or educational training for this purpose (BRASIL, 2005).

The availability of information can help parturients understand their rights and make them feel respected. In this sense, the contribution of health professionals goes beyond providing access to information and services. Some of the steps for carrying out humanized childbirth, which are considered to be parturients' rights, are: the presence of someone from the family to accompany the birth; receiving guidance on the birth and the procedures that will be adopted; freedom of movement during labor; the choice of position for the end of the birth; and relaxation to relieve pain and immediate mother-baby contact immediately after the birth. Respect for the parturient woman's wishes and rights is essential, including comfort, safety and well-being, as well as adequate pain control during labor and the presence of a companion chosen by the woman (CARVALHO *et al*, 2014).

According to Piccinini *et al* (2004), the new roles have only just been outlined and everything is still to be built and adapted to. The difficult task for parents-to-be essentially consists of the transition between being cared for and being a caregiver. And in order to accomplish this, they will need guidance. Success will depend on a number of factors, be they social, cultural or economic. Pregnancy serves as a period of preparation for the new roles that parents will have to take on in relation to the baby and everything it will require. These include fantasies and feelings, a review of their own childhood and parental roles, as well as the worries arising from this transition. This participation facilitates the formation of early bonds between parents and baby, strengthening family ties.

4.3 The Importance of Quality Prenatal Care

The Ministry of Health instituted the Prenatal and Birth Humanization Program (PHPN). Until then, there had been no model to standardize care for pregnant women in Brazil. This program established not only the number of consultations and the gestational age of entry, but also listed laboratory tests and health education actions, and brought about a discussion of health practices and their conceptual bases, in line with the models used around the world (FIGUEIREDO, 2011).

Quality prenatal care is fundamental to reducing maternal and perinatal mortality. Ensuring adequate care means preventing, diagnosing and treating undesirable events during pregnancy, with a view to the well-being of the pregnant woman and her unborn child, as well as providing guidance to avoid specific problems during childbirth, or even certain immediate care for the newborn (BRASIL, 2015).

An important part of humanizing childbirth is preparing the woman and her social network before the birth, so that she can know that childbirth is an event that depends primarily on her and the health team. They should be aware of their rights, such as: the right to a companion; the right to stay with their child immediately after delivery; labor rights; the right not to have a routine episiotomy; the right to privacy; the right to move around during labor; the right to choose when to allow vaginal touch, among many others (SPINELLI, 2008).

The clinical activity of prenatal care generally focuses on biological risks, exams and measurements. Most professionals, when in primary care, have very little willingness to carry out minimally adequate prenatal care, even nurses or doctors, find it difficult to carry out prenatal care beyond the physical examination, just as little is said to pregnant women about bodily changes, about sexuality, about exercises that prepare the perineum (and it's not enough to talk about it, you have to teach them how to do it), about non-pharmacological methods of pain relief (teaching massage to companions), about breathing, about fears, about family experience with childbirth, about preparing for other children, about what labor is and how it begins, about the postpartum period, about massages for the child, about visiting the health service where she will give birth, in short, losing the opportunity to exchange experiences and accounts of childbirth (BRASIL, 2015).

The obvious thing is that the more pregnancy is valued with all its meanings, the easier it is to diagnose organic problems when they occur, and the greater the involvement of women in treatment, so that instead of trying to subject women to cold and meaningless prenatal care, the humanization of prenatal care is demanding a leap in quality, This is an excellent time to build a network in defense of life and to improve maternal health and prevent avoidable deaths. It is also one of the objectives of greatest national and international interest in the field of reproductive health and rights, in which the necessary and effective measures to achieve this goal are being discussed (ANVERSA, 2012).

However, it is necessary to combine the security of obtaining good results with well-being for the woman and the newborn, while respecting their constitutional rights. In Brazil, care for women during pregnancy and childbirth remains a challenge, both in terms of quality itself and the philosophical principles of care, which are still centred on a medicalized, hospital-centred and technocratic model. Pregnant women's care is one of the longest-running activities in the country's public health services, and for many years it was mainly geared towards improving child health indicators (PETITO *et al*, 2015).

4. 4 The Role of Men in Childbirth

Reflections on the father's presence and participation in childbirth and postpartum, his role in the family context, and the baby's part in the formation of the new family, have led us to discuss what the real meaning of the father figure is and what changes might be taking place in the face of the diversity of family arrangements and the numerous socio-cultural contexts that converge (DA SILVA TARNOWSKIL; PRÓSPERO; ELSEN, 2005).

"The feminist movement of the 1960s, along with other social movements, was fundamental in changing the concept of the modern subject. The aim of this movement was equality in sexual difference. Claiming the non-hierarchical nature of the specificities of men and women, it sought a social equality that recognizes differences, today expressed in the notion of gender equality" (DA SILVA TARNOWSKIL; PRÓSPERO; ELSEN, 2005).

Internationally, research into masculinity emerged in the 1970s, but it was preceded by studies into women. In the following decade, studies on the social construction of masculinity appeared with greater consistency, directly benefiting from reflections on the concept of gender. Studies on paternity emerged as a particular field and investigated the more effective participation of men in everyday family life, more specifically in caring for children: this man came to be characterized as the new father (DA SILVA TARNOWSKIL; PRÓSPERO; ELSEN, 2005).

For Brazelton in 1988, there was already a new awareness that raising a child was also the father's job, but there was still no clarity about this new role, and the men who took on this responsibility did not always receive social support. Competition and exclusion were also frequent and expected feelings in future fathers, not only because the woman tends to divert her energies and attention to the baby, but also because she becomes the center of everyone's attention, and few are interested in the feelings of the future father during this period of adaptation. However, the man should make similar adaptations to the woman, and face similar doubts and anxieties (PICCININI *et al*, 2004).

In the 1990s, Maldonado, Dickstein and Nahoum (1997) pointed out that men's history of fatherhood is different from women's, since most fathers are unable to create solid bonds with their babies. It is only the mother who can feel the child grow, give birth and breastfeed it. At this time, the man is usually forgotten, few are interested in the feelings of the future father, where the baby and the mother become the center of attention. However, men also go through similar adaptations to women, and face similar doubts and anxieties. During pregnancy, paternal involvement must be understood in a special way, because the bond between father and child is indirect and can be mediated by the presence of the mother (PICCININI *et al*, 2004).

According to da Silva Tarnowskil; Próspero; Elsen (2005), the feminist movement generated many contradictions and brought about significant socio-economic and cultural changes. These were consolidated in the middle of the 20th century and led to changes in the conditions of women and men, triggering the need to seek different understandings of personal relationships and new family ties and configurations.

The great involvement of women in the professional field and the new social role of women's work, among other socio-economic factors, have opened up spaces for fathers to take part in caring for their children. In this way, fathers would be more active in their parenting, exerting direct influences on their children's development (PICCININI; BONILHA, 2004).

4. 5 Context Man vs. Woman

Until recently, being a father was a matter of course, and science and popular belief didn't attach much importance to the father's active participation during the child's development process. Pointing out that our society is going through a crisis of undefined social roles, it is necessary to reconstruct the role of men/fathers so that they can assume their own masculinity, exercising paternity and being able to make use of affection. The rapid rise in the number of separations/divorces and the removal of fathers from the family context inaugurated a strand of research that began to investigate the consequences of paternal absence. However, it wasn't until studies on women, driven by the feminist movement, that researchers sought to better understand masculinity and paternity, which came to be seen in a different light, as social constructs. Paternal involvement is more complex than it appears to be, especially in the phase following the birth of a child, when routines are abruptly changed (DA SILVA TARNOWSKIL; PRÓSPERO; ELSEN, 2005).

"The ideological updating of the genders, in the figure of the "new independent woman", makes it possible to hide the double working day, the exploitation and the way in which these strategies contribute to the reproduction of gender and social class inequality. It should be noted that this double working day is not a source of financial independence or even family stability. On the contrary, although it is necessary for the survival and upkeep of children, it is closely related to the breakdown of the male breadwinner in the context of unemployment and inadequate salaries to maintain a family. This male failure can result in male behaviors of giving up, panic and flight" (DA SILVA TARNOWSKIL; PRÓSPERO; ELSEN, 2005).

According to Motta and Crepaldi (2005), today, mothers work outside the home (and most of them work double shifts, i.e. professional and domestic work) and fathers take on domestic responsibilities for their children, such as day-to-day care. These changes are still shaping a new father. With the integration of men into labor, accompanying and comforting women is a new role for them. How he experiences this care depends on the possibilities of each father, the relationship between the couple and the expectations of both men and women at this time. It is necessary to consider that, just like the pregnant woman, the father-to-be is going through a process of adaptation and readjustment in order to experience fatherhood as a moment of transition that will allow for emotional growth.

In the 1980s, Soifer pointed out that men were in some way overwhelmed by the experience of pregnancy and the way in which they experienced this period could influence the way they deal with the situation during labor. It's worth pointing out that labor involves all those who accompany it, in a process of emotional intensity. In this way, men, as the woman's parents and partners, experience this moment with all the emotional burden (MOTTA; CREPALDI, 2005).

According to Tomeleria *et al* (2007), with the birth of a baby comes the formation of a family, allowing for a variety of arrangements, and it is necessary to think about the importance of the father's participation and his psycho-emotional context in the delivery and postpartum scene. This participation facilitates the formation of early bonds between father and baby, which aims to strengthen ties. For men, the process of giving birth can be a time of intense emotion, enabling the father's first direct contact with his child, without the intermediary of the mother, which is necessary during pregnancy, when the fetus is incorporated into the mother's body schema.

4. 6 The father as chaperone

By accompanying the birth of his child, the father creates bonds and is considered the ideal companion for the woman during labor, where the father is affirming his paternity and valuing his role. In this context, fathers cannot be denied the opportunity to experience one of the most important moments in a human being's life: birth. This would be the pinnacle of pregnancy for the father, as the baby becomes real to his new world and he can already carry it in his arms, which provides a bond of remarkable emotions (PERDOMINI; BONILHA, 2011).

According to da Silva Tarnowskil; Próspero; Elsen (2005), we understand that it is for these and many other reasons that the development of the human being, which begins with pregnancy and the whole process surrounding birth, must be rethought, starting with the inclusion of a relevant element: paternal participation.

According to the Ministry of Health, the humanization of care during birth and delivery is a current challenge and includes the inclusion of the father or companion of the parturient woman's choice. It requires that due attention be paid to the pregnant woman's perspective, as meeting her needs is a basic prerequisite of obstetric care. The father's active participation in the pregnancy is considered important, since it is believed that this attitude should be the result of a conscious decision made together with the pregnant woman, and not the result of a desire to meet the expectations of other family members, professionals and society itself (MAZZIERI; HOGA, 2006).

"The World Health Organization recommends that parturients should be accompanied by people they trust and with whom they feel comfortable, which could be their partner, their best friend, a doula or a nurse-midwife" (BRUGGEMANN; OSIS; PARPINELI, 2007).

Law No. 11.108, of April 7, 2005, obliges health services in the public network or those affiliated with the Unified Health System (SUS) to allow the presence of a companion chosen by the parturient throughout the period of labor, delivery and puerperium. Choosing the support of the child's father during these events is one of the proposals for humanizing care (TOMELERIA *et al*, 2007).

With the effective participation of the father in the delivery and postpartum process, the law is not only being complied with and respected, but it is also leveraging the relationship between the companion, the parturient woman and the professionals involved in the care, contributing to a positive experience throughout the pregnancy (BRUGGEMANN; OSIS; PARPINELI, 2007).

According to Tomeleria *et al* (2007), the monitoring of pregnant women during prenatal care and the set of attitudes towards pregnancy is part of a new behavior that men are seeing when it comes to fatherhood. Men have shown a greater interest in participating on a daily basis, expressed through companionship and caring for the pregnant woman and the child, training and adapting to fatherhood in a positive and full way.

Despite some changes already felt in the father-mother-child relationship, the exclusion of fathers from the reproductive health arena continues to occur in health programs. Rethinking this situation seems urgent in order to build gender equality in this field. With regard to childbirth, a moment when humanization includes, among other aspects, the presence of the father throughout the birth process. Empirically, what we can observe is that the presence of fathers in obstetric centers is still seen by professionals as disrupting routine activities. This also implies the father's passivity in the birth process. Therefore, without the proper reception and recognition of the importance of the father's presence in relieving the tensions of labour, whether caused by the physiology of childbirth or those related to the non-family environment, humanization cannot be achieved (TARNOWSKIL; PRÓSPERO; ELSEN, 2005).

5. 7 Psycho-emotional involvement

According to Piccinini *et al* (2004), paternal involvement in pregnancy highlights the fact that couples, and not just women, become pregnant, and that the changes that occur to fathers-to-be during pregnancy are not independent of the changes undergone by pregnant women themselves. Fathers can even develop Couvade's Syndrome, showing similar physical and psychological symptoms to women.

In this way, it is understood that fathers' involvement in pregnancy can be understood through their participation in activities related to pregnant women and preparations for the baby's arrival, the emotional support provided to the mother, the search for contact with the baby, as well as their worries and anxieties. However, according to the author, fathers differ considerably in the way they go through these stages, with some fathers not really being able to get involved with their child at any point during pregnancy (PICCININI *et al*, 2004).

Research has shown that the presence of a partner has a favorable influence on the progress of the pregnancy and reduces risks and unfavorable effects on the child's health, since insecurity and loneliness can cause physical and psychological risks. Support during and after childbirth favours the humanization of care, a reduction in unnecessary obstetric interventions and women's satisfaction with the birth experience (TOMELERIA *et al*, 2007).

Pregnancy is a new and intense event in a couple's life and is considered a unique experience. Childbirth is an explosion of feelings involving the family, especially the parents. It is a transitional phase, where feelings are mixed with anxiety and preparation for the birth of the baby, and new roles emerge. Each person can have multiple experiences and new sensations with the arrival of the new member, and it is necessary to work on their psycho-emotional reception so that they are ready for the changes, and that this special moment is pleasant and peaceful, contributing to a positive experience for both (PERDOMINI; BONILHA, 2011).

According to Piccinini *et al* (2004), the new roles have only just been outlined and everything has yet to be built and adapted. And in order to accomplish this, they will need guidance. Success will depend on a number of factors, be they social, cultural or economic. Pregnancy serves as a period of preparation for the new roles that parents will have to take on in the face of the baby and everything it will require. These include fantasies and feelings, a review of their own childhood and parental roles, as well as the worries arising from this transition. This participation facilitates the formation of early bonds between parents and baby, strengthening family ties.

5 METHODOLOGY

The methodology used in the research is presented below.

5. 1 Type of study

This is a qualitative, descriptive case study. The research requires a qualitative, descriptive approach, as the researcher seeks to reduce the distance between theory and data, between context and action, using the logic of phenomenological analysis, i.e. understanding phenomena by describing and interpreting them. In qualitative research, the social is seen as a world of meanings that is subject to investigation. It is the language of the social actors and their practices that are the raw materials of this approach. It is the level of meanings, motives, aspirations, attitudes, beliefs and values, expressed through common language and everyday life, that is the object of the qualitative approach (TEIXEIRA, 2001).

The case study is something special that is going to be researched, it is a personal investigation in which there is a look at people, offering an opportunity to present an aspect that has not yet been seen. It's not a problem, it's something that hasn't been sufficiently understood and you want to understand it.

5. 2 Inclusion criteria

The study included fathers (male) over the age of 18 who agreed to take part in the study.

5. 3 Exclusion Criteria

Fathers under the age of 18, and fathers who refused to take part in the research and who had not experienced the birth of their child.

5. 4 Research scenario

The study was carried out in the homes of parents who agreed to take part in the research.

5. 5 Population and Sample

The sample (five fathers) for the survey was selected on the recommendation of friends who had experienced the birth of their child and were willing to answer the questions about their experience of the pregnancy-puerperium cycle.

5. 6 Data Collection Instruments

An interview script was drawn up with the following variables: age, gender, occupation, number of pregnancies, and the object of the research: participation during pregnancy and childbirth, emotional aspects, experience, and the script with the following questions: What did you feel when you found out you were going to be a father?; What is it like to be a father?;

Why did you attend the birth?; Did your wife/partner/girlfriend/friend consent?; How did you participate in the stages of pregnancy?; Do you have more than one child? Was the emotion different? Describe your feelings during childbirth.

5. 7 Data collection

After presenting the research to the parents who were interviewed, they were invited to take part, and once they had accepted we asked them to sign the informed consent form (ICF), informing them that their identities would be preserved using pseudonyms. The data was collected between October and November 2015, according to the schedule.

6. 8 Ethical aspects

This study was evaluated by the Research Ethics Committee (CEP), and in accordance with the requirements of the Informed Consent Form (TCLE), it was approved under Resolution 466 of December 12, 2012. "This resolution incorporates, from the point of view of individuals and communities, the five basic references of bioethics: autonomy, non-maleficence, beneficence and justice and equity, among others, and aims to ensure the rights and duties that concern research participants, the scientific community and the State." Considering the respect for human dignity and the special protection of the lives of participants in scientific research involving human beings, it is resolved to comply with the following guidelines and norms:

a) In order to guarantee beneficence, we commit and assure the target informants of maximum benefit and minimum harm, both individual and collective, both actual and potential.

b) To ensure non-maleficence, we will assure the target informants that foreseeable harm will be avoided in cases of compensated harm.

c) In order to ensure fairness and equity, we emphasized to the target informants the social relevance of the reflections arising from the research, so that they could benefit from participating in it.

The pre-project was sent to the Research Ethics Committee (CEP) of the University of Amazonia via the Brazil platform, and after being approved the research began, respecting the cultural, social, religious and ethical values, as well as the habits and customs of the population being investigated. At the same time, the informed consent form (ICF) was requested and signed by the people involved in the research, guaranteeing the privacy and confidentiality of their names and the information provided during the stages of dissemination of the results.

The participants were informed individually, in clear and accessible language, about the aims of the research and the benefits it will provide, and that there will be no risks and no obligation to take part. They were also informed about the period during which their practices will be observed and the moments of conversation that will be used as interviews, where everyone was made aware that exclusion from the research could be requested at any time. In order to carry out this research, a time and place were scheduled for the interviews and observations, guaranteeing the right to privacy, with no exposure of the person or their information during or after the research. It was also explained that the information from this study will be used exclusively for scientific purposes in the fields of health and nursing.

5.9 Risks and benefits

5.9.1 Risks

The interview posed minimal physical and/or psychological risk to the interviewee. The names of the interviewees and the information provided were kept confidential, with privacy guaranteed by the researchers: Hisis da Costa Sousa, Jean Jorge da Silva Ferreira and Maria Luciana Olimpio Nascimento, for a period of five years, and incinerated after this period. The research subjects have been identified by pseudonyms.

5.9.2 Benefits

This research will contribute to forming a link between popular and scientific knowledge, thus enabling the community to get closer to the health services during maternity, which will reflect in a greater appreciation of the individual, bringing the family closer, strengthening the bonds between parents and children through respect for their beliefs and cultural habits.

5.10 Data Analysis

The data was analyzed using the content analysis method. Content analysis is a research methodology used to describe and interpret the content of all kinds of documents and texts pertinent to the subject being researched.

This analysis leads to systematic, qualitative or quantitative descriptions, as well as helping to reinterpret the messages and reach an understanding of their meanings at a level that goes beyond a common reading (BARDIN, 1979).

6 Results and discussion

The interviews were scheduled at a time desired by the interviewee and the preferred location was the home of each parent. They were carried out between September and October and there was no set time for each answer. The Terms of Free and Informed

Consent of the interviewee and the reporting forms were duly analyzed and signed by each collaborator. Some comments were made, but always avoiding influencing each interviewee's answers in any way. The questions were designed to explore the interviewee's expectations throughout the pregnancy up to the birth of the child, emphasizing their experience as a companion in this process of labor and birth. These answers were analyzed by reading each interview, punctuating each interviewee's decisions and views on the subject in paragraphs, and highlighting the most important phrases in each interview in quotation marks.

- How did you feel when you found out you were going to be a father?

"Fear! Being unemployed and a university student. Afraid of the changes that fatherhood would bring. I think I stopped feeling afraid after we told my partner's mother and mine. When we received support from family members, it was easier to let go of the fear and face up to the responsibilities."

(Bahia).

"As it was planned, the excitement only came afterwards, during the fittings and imaging tests." (Tocantins).

Men are identifying more and more with women, and have a desire to "mature", especially among young fathers. The "new father" who is emerging at the end of this century is a man who is trying to prepare himself emotionally to take on an active role in the care and upbringing of his children, just like his wife. The father feels just as responsible for his child as the mother and knows that it's not enough to see the child once in a while to be a good father (SANTO; BONILHA, 2000).

According to Gabriel and Dias (2011), for men, pregnancy and the birth of a child are crossed by different meanings that did not previously exist in their lives. Familiarity can generate countless feelings and particular ways of experiencing the arrival of the child, which can result in a confusion of feelings, mixing joy with sadness, and in the behaviors experienced by the father.

Discovering yourself as a father is an experience of new meanings, changes and responsibilities. It's something that involves expectations, dreams, fears and anxieties. For parents-to-be, the birth of a child marks an important transition in their lives. The baby, who is totally dependent, transforms the whole world around him or her, and the man and woman become father and mother. However, other functions and identities in their lives will have to adjust to these new roles. As a result, both men and women often have mixed feelings about having children, which can range from excitement at the news to feelings of anxiety and fear about the responsibility of caring for a child and the commitment of time and energy. For many men, feeling like a father is a fact that only occurs after the birth and, in some cases, even after the arrival of the child, the feeling of paternity is still not so recognizable, as is the weight of responsibility that this event presupposes.

- What does it mean to be a father?

"Being a father is much more than the person who pays the bills, it's the person who accompanies the development and stages of each child."

(Parà).

"Being a father is the greatest emotion a man can have, experiencing the purest and truest love"

(Tocantins).

In order for the man to become a father, he takes on both the model of fatherhood and the model of how a good father should be, in his own imagination. The man also suffers the impact of the change in roles. Fear, new feelings of love, and responsibility for the child can often lead men into a conflictual phase, where emotions are mixed with anxieties. And even then, the man doesn't stop questioning himself, both because of the previous generation and because of the demands of society. In taking this attitude, the man conceives a new and unique way of being a father, based on what he is experiencing at the moment - feelings, worries, expectations, doubts and the spaces that are being opened up for him to exercise his fatherhood in a natural and unique way (GABRIEL; DIAS, 2011).

The path towards becoming a father goes through the following stereotypes: having a child is a sign of masculinity; having a child means doing your job; the father is not needed in childbirth. The father has become the provider, he has stifled his emotions, he has stopped spending time with his children. Today, he wants to change that. He wants to be more present, participating, giving birth together with his wife, "fathering" (SANTO; BONILHA, 2000).

Fatherhood is built up little by little during pregnancy and can occur as men see their bellies grow. He needs to protect and be responsible for his children, taking part in their lives and, above all, looking after them. Becoming a father is a role that is undergoing a major transformation. We can see that a new attitude is being demanded of men, not only because of the stage of the life cycle they are entering, in which new functions are expected, but also because of society and especially the media, which is demanding that men be closer and more involved in family matters. It is no longer accepted that fathers only pay for their children's expenses, but that they have a duty to spend time with them, to take part in their upbringing and care, and to be emotionally available for them.

- Why attend childbirth?

"*I think my fear was always that I wouldn't be able to attend the birth because of some eventuality. The idea of not being next to my partner and being able to experience that moment scared me a lot.*"

(Bahia).

"*It was the right decision from the moment we decided we were going to be parents, because I would never miss the chance to take part in the most important moment of our lives and, I believe, of every couple's life.*"

(Cearà).

For the Brazilian Ministry of Health, which has established a care protocol indicating the need for the parturient woman to have a companion of her choice as part of the humanization of childbirth care, it is the target of attention from professionals and those responsible for proposing public policies at international level. It includes the inclusion of a companion of the parturient woman's choice (although this recommendation has not yet been incorporated into the daily practice of many Brazilian institutions), who is generally excluded from the birth and delivery process (HOGA; PINTO, 2007).

This research shows through the fathers' own testimonies that this clientele is increasingly committed to participating and actively accompanying the woman in the puerperal pregnancy cycle, and it is such a dependency that it makes the father almost obligatory as the best option for companionship at this time. The answers to this question are justified by the enthusiasm of the majority of the fathers (who could never physically express their happiness in words) who said that "they would never miss one of the happiest moments of their lives" and that it would be the end of an entire journey that began with the first steps in prenatal consultations and examinations such as ultrasound, where they were most excited.

Accompanying fathers at all stages of pregnancy is becoming a modern trend, as it is an early and positive way of strengthening the relationship between father and child, which begins mainly at the moment of birth and will last a lifetime. Other fathers reported that they wanted to take part because they wanted to protect mother and child, and also because they were curious about the long-awaited moment of seeing their child for the first time.

- Has the wife, partner, girlfriend, friend consented to the partner or husband attending the birth?

"Yes. Not just at the birth, but at every stage of the pregnancy, I was there" (Parà).

"Yes. It was our decision, where she would feel safer" (Piaui).

The answer was unanimously yes. Even with fear and many doubts at this time, there is still a concern on the part of the father to make a point of participating in a significant way in the child's birth, as some reported that it was the father's wish, others the couple's and in some cases a request from the mother herself, as she believes that she will be better protected with her husband present.

Other parents were restless and worried about the delay in giving birth and uncomfortable in the delivery room, both because it was an unfamiliar environment and because they were afraid of being taken away at any moment, even though some of them knew about the law on companions, they were afraid

that they would be ignored and in any case prevented from attending the birth of the child who would be the happiest at that moment.

The act of accompanying the birth becomes a law and the exclusive right of the parturient to authorize who she wants to be with her at that moment is not the exclusive role of the father, if she doesn't authorize it, because she is protected by Law no. 11.108, of April 7, 2005, which obliges health services in the public network or those affiliated to the Unified Health System (SUS), to authorize the presence of a companion chosen by the parturient, throughout the period of labour, delivery and puerperium, with the choice of support from the child's father during these events, as one of the proposals for humanizing care (BRASIL, 2005).

- How did you participate in the pregnancy?

"I was there for every part of the process. I followed the consultations and every development of the pregnancy. I interacted and shared with my partner about every new development in my son's life."

(Bahia).

"I've always taken part: I've witnessed all the nausea, I've been to all the appointments, the ultrasounds, we read stories and sang while my daughter was in her belly, I helped with the layette, I looked for information about pregnancy and childbirth, I took part in everything."

(Piaui).

Paternal involvement in pregnancy doesn't just refer to behaviors such as going to appointments and ultrasound scans. It also refers to emotional involvement, and these aspects are not necessarily related (MAY, 1982). In this way, it is understood that fathers' involvement in pregnancy can be understood through their participation in activities related to pregnant women and preparations for the baby's arrival, the emotional support provided to the mother, the search for contact with the baby, as well as their worries and anxieties (PICINNI, 2004).

We can see from the answers above to the question: how did you participate in the pregnancy? All the fathers in this survey described that they participated effectively in all the stages of pregnancy, going to all the prenatal appointments, ultrasounds, helping with the nausea, reading and singing to the baby when it was still in the mother's belly, helping with the baby's trousseau and room, as well as seeking more information about pregnancy and childbirth, and these fathers also described the emotional support, comfort and security for their partners.

- Do you have more than one child? Was the emotion different? Describe your emotions during childbirth.

"*The emotion can't be described in words, there's nothing like it, no matter how many achievements I've had in my life."*

(Tocantins).

"I felt very tired, very tired! I needed to help her with the exercises that would make the birth easier. At the time of the birth, I remember feeling very happy, anxious and curious. Happiness at knowing that we had managed to have our humanized home birth, anxiety at knowing what my son would do and how we would react. Curiosity to see his face.

(Bahia).

"I felt really good! All my fears and anxieties about the future disappeared during the time I was in the delivery room, and especially when I saw my daughter's face and held her in my arms for the first time."

(Piaui).

"I have two children. The emotion was the same, but with less nervousness. An indescribable feeling.

(Parà).

The way paternity is experienced is changing and the father's participation in the delivery room is under construction. However, the most important thing to consider is that the father is emotionally involved in the birth and, symbolically, giving birth together with the woman. This experience can result in fathers who are more committed to their family's health and quality of life (TOMELERI, *et al* 2007).

The fathers interviewed described their feelings during childbirth as moments of great expectation and as unique experiences in their lives, where they reported difficulty in describing in words, but some gave more details and others did not, of this feeling during childbirth. And of these parents, only one has two children, where he described that the emotion was the same as less nervousness. As we can see from the parents' answers to the question: do you have more than one child? Was the emotion different? Describe your emotions during childbirth.

Research shows that, for men, childbirth is a time of intense emotion, enabling the first direct contact between the father and the child, without the intermediation of the woman, which is necessary during pregnancy, when the fetus is incorporated into the mother's body schema. Furthermore, when the father participates emotionally in the birth of his child, this fact, in a way, helps to restore and reinforce the couple's integration (DAVIM, MENEZES, 2001).

And as we can also see in the answers from the fathers from Tocantins, Bahia and Piaui above, all the fathers were present from the moment of childbirth to the end, where these fathers recount their anxieties, fears, tiredness and, above all, the emotion of being able to witness the long-awaited birth and seeing their children's faces, putting an end to all the anxiety of knowing what they would be like when they looked at and held their children for the first time. All the fathers showed their dedication to being a father and said that these were the greatest and best moments of their lives, moments they would never forget.

7 FINAL CONSIDERATIONS

The path we used to study the psycho-emotional aspects of fathers during the pregnancy-puerperium cycle enabled us to study issues peculiar to men in the context of being fathers. Fatherhood can be experienced by men who love, who are emotional, who are sensitive, who suffer and who take pleasure in experiencing childbirth. Today's man wants to be present throughout the pregnancy, he wants to be a father at the same time as his wife becomes a mother, staying by her partner's side and helping to give birth to the child that belongs to both of them.

Fathers are considered to be the ideal companions for women during childbirth, since accompanying the birth of their child means that they are realizing their paternity, valuing their role and strengthening family ties. The fathers interviewed were able to take part in all stages of pregnancy, childbirth and the postpartum period of their own volition and that of their partners, as well as being supported by Law No. 11.108, of April 7, 2005, or the law on companionship.

The high incidence of emotional involvement reported by the fathers in the survey is related to fear, anxiety, distress, insecurity, emotion of various aspects and curiosity, especially in seeing their child's face. Observing both emotional and behavioral involvement, these data reveal indications of a profound change in parenthood during pregnancy.

Hospital institutions must ensure compliance with the law, which guarantees the presence of a companion of the woman's choice during the birth process, since the father cannot be denied one of the most exciting moments in the couple's lives: birth.

In this sense, nursing has an important role to play in proposing and maintaining projects to include companions in childbirth care. Great importance has been attached to the fact that this professional prepares the companion for active participation in childbirth. In addition to the fact that the companion plays a fundamental role as a facilitator and promoter of the understanding of the needs evidenced in care, we hope that this research will contribute to the teaching and research perspectives for health professionals and parents who are looking for this topic, contributing to improving care in health practices.

REFERENCES

ANVERSA, Elenir Terezinha Rizzettiet *al.* **Quality of the prenatal care process: basic health units and Family Health Strategy units in a municipality in southern Brazil**. Cad saùde pùblica, v. 28, n. 4, p. 789-800, 2012. Available at: http://www.scielo.br/pdf/csp/v28n4/18.pdf. Accessed on: April 20, 2015.

BARDIN, L. **Content analysis**. Sâo Paulo: Altas. 1979.

BRANDÂO, Sónia Maria Pereira de Azevedo. **Fathers' emotional involvement with their babies: the impact of the childbirth experience.** 2009. Master's Degree in Nursing Sciences. Abel Salazar Institute of Biomedical Sciences.

University of Porto, Portugal, 2009. Available at:

http://repositorio.chporto.pt/bitstream/10400.16/1384/1/Sonia%20Brandao%20%20Dissertacao.pdf. Accessed on: April 15, 2015.

BRAZIL. Law No. 11.108, of April 7, 2005. Amends Law No. 8.080, of September 19, 1990, to guarantee parturients the right to have a companion present during labor, delivery and the immediate postpartum period, within the scope of the Unified Health System - SUS. **Official Journal of the Union**. Brasilia; 2005 [cited 2011 Apr 4]. Available at: http://www.planalto.gov.br/ccivil_03/_Ato2004-2006/2005/Lei/L11108.htm. Accessed on: April 17, 2015.

BRAZIL. Law No. 8080, of September 19, 1990. Provides for the conditions for the promotion, protection and recovery of health, the organization and operation of the corresponding services and other measures. **Official Gazette** of **the Union of** 1999; September 20. Available at: http://www.planalto.gov.br/ccivil_03/leis/L8080.htm.

Accessed on: April 20, 2015.

BRAZIL. Law No. 9.263, of January 12, 1996. Regulates § 7 of Art. 226 of the Federal Constitution, which deals with Family Planning, establishes penalties and makes other provisions. **Official Gazette of the Federative Republic of Brazil.** Brasilia, January 15, 1996. Section: 01. Available:

http://www.planalto.gov.br/ccivil_03/Leis/L9263.htm. Accessed on: 17 Apr. 2015.

BRUGGEMANN, Odaléa Maria; OSIS, Maria José Duarte; PARPINELLI, Mary Angela. **Support at birth: perceptions of professionals and companions chosen by the woman**. Rev Saùde Pùblica, v. 41, n. 1, p. 44-52, 2007. Available: http://www.scielosp.org/pdf/rsp/v41n1/5409.pdf. Accessed on: 30 abri. 2015.

CARVALHO, Vanessa Franco de *et al.* **Rights of parturients: knowledge of adolescents and companions**. Saùde e Sociedade, v. 23, n. 2, p. 572-581, 2014. Available at: http://www.revistas.usp.br/sausoc/article/download/84890/87626. Accessed on: April 17, 2015.

DA SILVA TARNOWSKI, Karina; PRÓSPERO, Elisete Navas Sanches; ELSEN, Ingrid. **Paternal participation in the process of humanizing birth: a question to be rethought**. Texto & Contexto Enfermagem, v. 14, p. 103-108, 2005. Available at: http://www.scielo.br/pdf/tce/v14nspe/a12v14nspe.pdf. Accessed on: May 7, 2015.

DAVIM, Rejane Marie Barbosa; DE MENEZES, Rejane Maria Paiva. Assistance to normal childbirth at home. **Revista Latino-Americana de Enfermagem**, v. 9, n. 6, p. 62-68, 2001. Accessed on 06/11/2015 at 14hrs.

ESPIRITO SANTO, Lilian Cordova do; BONILHA, Ana Lùcia de Lourenzi. **Expectations, feelings and experiences of fathers during childbirth**. *Revista gaùcha de enfermagem. Porto Alegre. Vol. 21, n. 2 (jul. 2000), p. 87-109,* 2000. Available:

http://www.lume.ufrgs.br/bitstream/handle/10183/23477/000290002.pdf?sequence=1 . Accessed on: 05 Nov. 2015.

FIGUEIREDO, Bàrbara; COSTA, Raquel; PACHECO, Alexandra. **Childbirth experience: Some factors and associated consequences**. Anàlise Psicològica, v. 20, n. 2, p. 203-217, 2012. Disponivelem: http://publicacoes.ispa.pt/index.php/ap/article/view/306/pdf. Accessed: Apr. 21, 2015.

GABRIEL, Marilia Reginato; DIAS, Ana Cristina Garcia. **Perceptions of fatherhood: describing oneself and one's father as a father**. *Estudpsicol (Natal)*, 2011, 16.3: 253-61. Available: http://www.scielo.br/pdf/epsic/v16n3/07.pdf. Accessed on: 05 Nov. 2015.

HOGA, Luiza AkikoKomura, and Cleusa Maia de Souza PINTO. **"Childbirth care with the presence of a companion: experiences of professionals."***Investigación y educaciónenfermeria* 25.1 (2007): 74-81.

LEITE, ACNMT *et al*. **Women's rights in Brazil: a focus on maternal health**. História, Ciências, Saùde-Manguinhos, Rio de Janeiro, v. 16, n. 3, p. 705 714, 2009. Available at: http://www.scielo.br/pdf/hcsm/v16n3/08.pdf. Accessed on: April 15, 2015.

MAZZIERI, Silvia Patricia Madureira; HOGA, Luiza AkikoKomura. **Father participation in birth and delivery: a literature review**. Revista Mineira de Enfermagem, v. 10, n. 2, p. 166-170, 2006. Available: http://www.reme.org.br/artigo/detalhes/402. Accessed on: May 27, 2015.

MOTTA, Cibele Cunha Lima da. CREPALDI, Maria Aparecida. **The father in childbirth and emotional support: The perspective of the parturient**. Paidéia. V.15, n. 30, p. 105-118, 2005. Available: http://www.scielo.br/pdf/paideia/v15n30/12.pdf. Accessed on April 13, 2015.

NASCIMENTO, Keyla Cristiane do *et al*. **The art of midwifery: care experience of traditional midwives in Envira/AM**. Escola Anna Nery Revista de Enfermagem, v. 13, n. 2, p. 319-327, 2009. Available at: http://www.scielo.br/pdf/ean/v13n2/v13n2a12.pdf. Accessed on: 17 Apr. 2015.

OLIVEIRA, Eteniger Marcela Fernandes de. **Men's experience of the puerperium**. 2007. Available at: http://repositorio.ufrn.br:8080/jspui/bitstream/123456789/14637/1/EtenigerMFO.pdf. Accessed on: April 15, 2015.

OSAWA, Ruth Hitomi; RIESCO, Maria Luiza Gonzales; TSUNECHIRO, Maria Alice. **Midwives-nurses and nurse-midwives: the interface of related but distinct professions**. RevBrasEnferm, v. 59, n. 5, p. 699-702, 2006. Available at: http://www.scielo.br/pdf/reben/v59n5/v59n5a20.pdf. Accessed on: April 15, 2015.

PERDOMINI, Fernanda Rosa Indriunas; BONILHA, Ana L. cia de Lourenzi. **The participation of fathers as companions during childbirth**. Texto e Contexto Enfermagem, v. 20, n. 3, p. 245, 2011. Available at:

http://www.scielo.br/pdf/tce/v20n3/04.pdf. Accessed on: Apr. 19, 2015.

PETITO, Anamaria Donato Castro *et al.* **The importance of father participation in the puerperal pregnancy cycle: a literature review**. REFACER-Revista Eletrônica da Faculdade de Ceres, v. 1, n. 4, 2015. Available at:

http://ceres.facer.edu.br/revista/index.php/refacer/article/view/70/46. Accessed on: 15 Apr. 2015.

PICCININI, Cesar Augusto *et al.* **Paternal involvement during pregnancy**. Psicologia: Reflexao e Critica, v. 17, n. 3, p. 303-314, 2004. available at

http://www.scielo. br/pdf/prc/vl 7n3⁄a03v17n3. Accessed on April 20, 2015.

REIS, Adriana Elias dos; PATRICIO, Zuleica Maria. **Application of the actions recommended by the Ministry of Health for humanized childbirth in a hospital in Santa Catarina**.Ciênc. saùde coletiva, Rio de Janeiro, v. 10, supl. p. 221-230, dez. 2005. Available available at

<http://www.scielosp.org/scielo.php?script=sci_arttext&pid=S141381232005000500023&lng=pt&nrm=iso>. Accessed on: April 20, 2015.

RIOS, Isabel Cristina. **Humanization: the essence of technical and ethical action in health practices**. RevBraseducméd, v. 33, n. 2, p. 253-62, 2009. Available at: http://www.scielo.br/pdf/rbem/v33n2/13.pdf. Accessed on: April 25, 2015.

SERRUYA, Suzanne Jacob; LAGO, Tânia Di Giàcomo; CECATTI, José Guilherme. **The panorama of prenatal care in Brazil and the Prenatal and Birth Humanization Program**. Rev. bras. saùde matern. infant, v. 4, n. 3, p. 269-279, 2004. Available at: http://www.scielo.br/scielo.php?script=sci_arttext&pid=S1519- 38292004000300007. Accessed on: April 17, 2015.

SILVA, Larissa Mandarano da; BARBIERI, Màrcia; FUSTINONI, Suzete Maria. **Experiencing childbirth in a humanized care model**. Rev. bras. enferm, v. 64, n. 1, p.

60-65, 2009. Available at: http://www.scielo.br/scielo.php?script=sci_arttext&pid=S0034-71672011000100009.

Accessed on: April 17, 2015.

SPINELLI, Maria Benita *et al.* **Humanized Attention to Women in the Pregnancy-Puerperium Cycle: Obstetrics Agenda**. Secretary of Health - Recife, 2008. Available at: http://www.recife.pe.gov.br/noticias/arquivos/1144.pdf. Accessed on: April 21, 2015.

TEIXEIRA, Elizabeth. **The three methodologies: academic, science and research.** 5th edition, Petrópolis- RJ: Contexto, 2001. 123 p. Available: http://bases.bireme.br/cgi-bin/wxislind.exe/iah/online/?IsisScript=iah/iah.xis&src.

Accessed on: April 21, 2015.

TOMELERI, Keli Regiane *et al.* **"I saw my son born": parents' experiences in the delivery room**. Revista Gaùcha de Enfermagem, v. 28, n. 4, p. 497, 2007.

Available: http://www.seer.ufrgs.br/RevistaGauchadeEnfermagem/article/view/3110/0. Accessed on: 13 Apr. 2015.

CHAPTER IV - THE MEANING OF HUMANIZATION: THE VOICE OF NEONATOLOGY NURSES IN PARA.

ANA CAROLINA DA SILVA

LUARA LETiCIA ASSUNÇÂO DE SALES

MARIA ALICE MONTEIRO PADILHA

MARCELO WILLIAMS OLIVEIRA DE SOUZA

SUMMARY

In modern society, with the advance of technology, human beings end up, even if unthinkingly, practicing dehumanization to the point of objectifying people and deifying technology. And one way to soften the harshness of this reality is to rediscover humanization. Nurses as mediators, regardless of the unit they work in, carry out interdisciplinary activities, always focusing on the care and safety of their clients, with a view to effectiveness and efficiency. Thus, the nurse who works in the neonatal intensive care unit must develop the skills necessary for excellent care and management, extending them beyond technical knowledge, reinforcing behavioral skills and attitudes that subtly differentiate truly competent and humanized care, thus providing holistic nursing care in order to improve care in the unit. Based on this, we will carry out a qualitative study of a descriptive nature with nurses who work in the Neonatal Intensive Care Unit at a reference hospital in Belém, Parà, Brazil, with the aim of understanding the meaning of humanization for each one, by means of an interview consisting of questions directed at the topic. Based on Bardin's theory.

Key words: Humanization, ICU, Neonatology.

1 INTRODUCTION

1.1 TOPIC UNDER STUDY

This study addresses the meaning of humanization for neonatal ICU nurses. According to the Ministry of Health (2013) in this context, we understand that humanization should be included in all areas and stages of the management and care process and put into practice not in isolation, but in a shared and collective way, being included as a new model of care.

While the organization and functioning of health systems in the 1980s was marked by the principles of effectiveness, optimization and efficiency, the 1990s saw the incorporation of the notions of quality, equity, satisfaction and user autonomy. This is where the humanization of health care comes in (FONTES, 2004).

Fontes (2004) says that in health care, humanizing means understanding each person in their singularity, taking into account their values and experiences without any form of discrimination, respecting and preserving their dignity.

Humanizing refers to the possibility of a cultural transformation of the management and practices developed in health institutions, assuming an ethical stance of respect for the other, of welcoming the unknown, of respect for the user understood as a citizen and not just as a consumer of health services (FONTES, 2004).

Based on the Universal Declaration of Human Rights, art. 1: "All human beings are born free and equal in dignity and rights. Endowed with reason and conscience, they should act towards one another in a spirit of brotherhood" (SOUZA; FERREIRA, 2008).

In recent years, initiatives to humanize care have been proposed with the importance of combining techniques and technologies. With the aim of better patient care. Today, humanization initiatives are present in various fields of care, but were initially implemented in childbirth and newborn care (SOUZA; FERREIRA, 2008).

The National Hospital Humanization Program - PNHAH, was instituted by the Ministry of Health, through Ordinance No. 881, of 06/19/2001, within the scope of the Unified Health System (BRASIL, 2002). The PNHH aims to implement the humanization project by improving care and the bond between patient, professional and family.

Based on the idea that the Intensive Care Unit is for critically ill patients who are more likely to recover, professionals seek to maximize their chances of living longer and better with quality, humanized care (SALICIO; GAIVA, 2006).

According to Reichert (2006) "The child is a unique being, full of potentialities, experienced throughout its intrauterine life". The Neonatal Intensive Care Unit (NICU) provides a totally different environment from the uterine environment. In this context, the Intensive Care Center (ICU) has brought to the Newborn (NB) a wide range of assistance, allowing the survival of those babies who would have had little chance of survival.

With this care and measures, they provide the best growth and development of the NB, achieving a satisfactory recovery and helping to minimize the effects of hospitalization, making parents active elements in the quality and survival of the patient (REICHERT; COLLET, 2006).

The ICU, in turn, is an environment with bright lights and constant noise, sometimes with interruptions to the sleep cycle, changes in temperature, assessments, procedures, all of which bring discomfort and pain to the NB. This brings with it the need to humanize the environment together - nursing professional, patient and mother (REICHERT; COLLET, 2006).

Some measures should be taken to humanize care, such as (REICHERT; COLLET, 2006).

The Kangaroo Mother Method, originally proposed by Dr. Edgar Rey Sanabria at the Maternal and Child Institute (IMI) in Bogotà, Colombia, in 1978 and adapted to the Brazilian reality in 2002, is an example of the implementation of the humanized care model in the neonatal field. This method promotes humanized care for low-birth-weight newborns and generates a set of care actions involving the patient, their family and health professionals (SOUZA; FERREIRA, 2008).

On the other hand, the nursing team also has to deal with death, which is where the anguish of the patient's suffering comes from, and if not dealt with properly, can cause stress, psychic suffering, which ends up being enhanced by the way the situation is dealt with, with nurses often making their care mechanized and inhumane. In order to achieve humanized care, it is necessary for humanization to be the institution's philosophy (OLIVEIRA, 2006).

Based on this, in order to achieve good professional care for newborns, it is necessary to include the family. The aim is to train professionals to have an interpersonal relationship based on human rights so that their work is based on humanized health care (COLLET, 2006).

1.2 BACKGROUND

Pregnancy is a very special time for a woman and, when she is about to "give birth", she becomes insecure and anxious, waiting for her baby to be born so that she can breastfeed him and give him enough care. However, due to something that happened during the birth, the baby needs to be taken to the Intensive Care Unit and this admission to the ICU sometimes abruptly breaks the possible reality in which the mother and her family were expecting the birth of a healthy baby. The ICU, on the other hand, cares for critically ill patients with conditions or illnesses that expose them to high risks, but which are more likely to recover. Because it is an environment in which the risk of death is eminent, it requires nurses to acquire skills, abilities, attitudes, dynamism, maturity, emotional balance and humanization. Based on this, what instigated us to research the meaning of humanization for neonatal ICU nurses was the fact that, regardless of age, newborns are also capable of expressing feelings, from the most pleasant to the most painful, and because the ICU is a sector in which the family feels it is an environment of suffering, professionals must take care to provide both the patient and their family with humanistic care, promoting well-being and reducing the degree of stress for both. Humanizing is nothing more than making care human so that you can take a holistic approach to your patient.

1.3 PROBLEMATICS AND GUIDING QUESTIONS

The ICU is considered to be a closed environment with excessive workloads, emergency situations, occupational risks and conflicting interpersonal relationships, which end up causing the team stress, leading to physical and mental exhaustion. As a result of these interferences, professionals end up changing their attitudes, both within the family and within the hospital, compromising the quality of their work and client care, with consequences for patients and their families (PEREIRA; MIRANDA; PASSOS, 2009).

Given the stress, lack of patience and double working hours, nurses end up making their care mechanized, and even unthinkingly turning it into dehumanized care.

Therefore, it is necessary to know, what is the purpose of identifying its flaws and if necessary improving them, hence we instigated the research on **THE SIGNIFICANCE OF HUMANIZATION: VOICE OF NEONATOLOGIST NURSES IN PARA?**

The following guiding questions also emerged:

a) What are nurses' perceptions of humanization in the NICU?

b) Is there a newborn care protocol?

c) The existence of SAE in the NICU?

d) The presence of psycho-social support for RNS mothers?

1.4 OBJECTIVES

1.4.1 General Objective

- Understanding the meaning of humanization among nurses working in the Neonatal ICU.

1.4.2 Specific Objectives

- Investigate the existence of a newborn care protocol.
- To investigate the existence of the nursing care system in the NICU.
- Identify the presence of psycho-social support for mothers of NBs.

2 THEORETICAL FRAMEWORK

2.1 Ethics

Ethics aims to understand the criteria and values that guide the judgment of human action in its many activities, especially those that concern work and associated human life (PINTO, 2008).

When one chooses a job as a profession, it needs to be something stimulating that leads the professional, on their own, to carry out tasks not just because they chose it, but because they identify with it. (SA, 2005)

2.2 Tertiary care

According to Potter Perry (2012), tertiary care is focused on intensive and sub-acute care and therefore requires increased assistance.

2.3 Intensive Care Unit

Potter Perry (2012) describes the ICU as a hospital unit in which the client receives monitoring and intensive care.

2.4 Psychological Practice in the Neonatal Intensive Care Unit

Hospital psychology is directly linked to the knowledge of psychology, which aims to detect and interfere in psychological issues related to illness, treatment and hospitalization in order to promote and/or recover the mental health of patients, families and the multidisciplinary team. Because the ICU is imagined as a frightening environment, feelings of fear and uncertainty are intensified, which is why the attention of a professional psychologist is necessary, justified by the "psychological urgency" in which patients and their families find themselves (REICHERT; COLLET, 2006).

The birth of a baby requires a certain psychic reorganization of roles for all the members of a family. Despite all the changes, the normal birth of a child is synonymous with celebration for everyone, both the family and the medical team. However, plans and expectations don't always turn out as expected, such as the birth of a premature baby or a baby with serious illnesses or malformations. This makes it necessary to hospitalize the newborn in the neonatal ICU, which is treated by the mother and family members as a moment of crisis, revealing a reality far removed from the idealized one.

The separation of mother and baby is abrupt and disrupts various psychic representations of this encounter (REICHERT; COLLET, 2006).

2.5 Structure and Organization of the Neonatal ICU

In order to talk about the structure and organization of a neonatal ICU, it is necessary to take into account the technological and therapeutic advances aimed at assisting high-risk neonates. All planning must be geared towards caring for the newborn and the family, from admission to discharge. Organization must be necessary, from the choice of equipment to human resources (TOMEZ; SILVA. Pg, 01, 2006).

The structure of the hospital where the neonatal ICU will be located must ensure that it has all the technical and human resources to meet the demands of caring for the sick newborn 24 hours a day, such as: (TOMEZ; SILVA. 2006)

- Clinical Laboratory, Pathological Laboratory, Radiology, Pharmacy, ECG, Social Services, Echocardiogram, Blood Gas, Blood Bank.

1.1.1 The Look of the Nurse on Duty

According to Tomez and Silva (2006), nurses are responsible for:

- Distributing the team's daily tasks.
- Receiving the shift together with the team, taking note of events such as the general condition of the patients, radiological and laboratory examinations (carried out and to be carried out), special care, medication, nutrition, vital signs, participation of parents, etc.
- Planning and prescribing nursing care for patients.
- Collaborate with the team in caring for the most serious patients.
- Supervising and coordinating transfers within the unit.
- Supervising nursing staff. Preparing and administering: blood and blood derivatives, strictly dosed drugs such as digitalis, psychotropic drugs, vasopressors, antiarrhythmics, heparin, insulin, etc.
- Supervising the installation of equipment such as mechanical ventilators.
- Collaborate with the nursing and medical team in procedures such as endotracheal intubation, umbilical catheterization, exsanquine transfusion, vein dissection, peripheral percutaneous catheter placement.
- Coordinating the nursing team in cardiac arrest care.
- Put the times on the doctor's prescriptions.
- Reviewing medical and nursing prescriptions, as well as nursing reports, in order to check that treatments and care have been carried out.
- Perform nasogastric, orogastric and bladder catheterization if necessary.
- Assisting the nursing team in performing endotracheal tube and upper airway aspiration.
- Performing venipunctures.
- Handle and control the equipment in the sector, keeping it ready for use.
- Keeping the unit manager informed of any problems with equipment that needs repairing or replacing, as well as the stock of materials.
- Collaborating with the sector's management in drawing up routine actions.
- Substitute for the unit manager in his/her absence.

- Maintain open communication with the patient's parents, evaluating the service, their concerns, needs and dissatisfaction with the service.
- Collaborate with the unit manager in research, training and continuing education programs.
- Participate in intra-hospital transport.
- Participate in the care of newborns at high-risk births.
- Maintain strict control of narcotics and drugs when receiving and passing on the plant.
- Maintaining a good relationship with the hospital's other sectors and departments; informing the manager of any abnormalities.
- Complying with and enforcing the hospital's general regulations, the regulations of the nursing department and the routines and regulations of the neonatal ICU.

2.6 History of Neonatology

Oliveira (2005) states that during the 19th century, care for newborns and children was carried out by foundations dedicated to caring for them because they were ignored by the medical profession in conjunction with institutions, and because of this, the mortality rate at that time was high. Hence, the process of transformation in neonatal care took place slowly, from the end of the 19th century to the beginning of the 20th century. Between 1870 and 1920, the European population contributed to the emergence of the Children's Health Movement, which sought to preserve the lives of premature infants and newborns, making it the milestone of neonatal medicine. At the end of the 19th century and the beginning of the 20th century, incubators were manufactured and maternity hospitals expanded to better treat newborns born with different illnesses; and in terms of prevention, prenatal care was developed. In the first half of the 20th century, several changes took place in childcare, especially for premature babies. At the same time, there were technological advances aimed at maintaining the lives of premature infants with respiratory problems.

Neonatal nursing in Brazil emerged predominantly focused on preventive actions, through charities and philanthropies, and in the mid-19th century social institutions were created to care for children (RODRIGUES, 2005).

2.7 Neonatal Epidemiology

The World Health Organization uses the infant mortality rate as a fundamental indicator for evaluating health care and the living conditions of a population. This coefficient is the ratio between the absolute number of deaths of children under one year of age, in a given place and period, and the total number of live births, in this same place and period, multiplied by 1,000. And for a better analysis of this data, the coefficient according to the period covered is as follows: (LACERDA, 2011)

- Early neonatal mortality (0 to 6 days of life).
- Late neonatal mortality (7 to 27 days of life).
- Post-neonatal mortality (28 to 364 days of life).

Over time, there has been a reduction in all three components of CMI in Brazil. In order to achieve a reduction in infant mortality, it is necessary to combine measures ranging from prenatal and childbirth care, to expanding the number of ICU beds and professionals trained to care for high-risk newborns (LACERDA, 2011).

2.8 Newborn Care Infrastructure

The infrastructure for newborn care, according to the standards of the Ministry of Health and the Neonatology Department of the Brazilian Society of Pediatrics, involves the following sectors (LACERDA, 2011).

- Delivery room:

Pediatric and nursing staff trained in neonatal resuscitation according to the updated standards of the Brazilian Society of Pediatrics.

- Co-housing:

It's a hospital system in which a healthy newborn baby, immediately after birth, remains by its mother's side 24 hours a day in the same environment until it is discharged from hospital.

- Kangaroo unit:

> The Kangaroo Mother Care Method is a type of neonatal care that involves early skin-to-skin contact between the mother and the low birth weight newborn, gradually and for as long as they both feel is pleasurable and sufficient, thus allowing the parents to participate more in the care of their newborn. (RODRIGUES. Pg. 17, 2011)

Early contact is done in a guided manner and is free for the family, accompanied by a properly trained health team. It takes place over three periods.

I. Period: during the newborn's stay in the intermediate and/or intensive care units.

II. Period: occurs after the newborn has stabilized, and the mother can stay with her child all the time in a joint ward, called the Kangaroo Unit.

III. Period: consists of monitoring the child in the outpatient clinic after discharge from hospital.

- Neonatal intermediate care unit:

Also known as the Medium Risk or Semi-Intensive Unit, it is the place where medium-risk newborns are cared for, such as those coming from the ICU; in the first 24 to 48 hours; in the first 72 hours of newborns weighing between 1,500 and 2,000 g; mild respiratory distress; need for venoclysis for glucose, electrolyte and antibiotic infusion; treatment of severe neonatal jaundice; premature infants gaining weight.

- Neonatal intensive care units:

It is designed to care for newborns with hemodynamic instability, severe metabolic disorders, respiratory failure, altered vital functions, weighing less than 1,200 g, requiring parenteral nutrition, central catheterization, surgery and other life-threatening patients. They must have uninterrupted medical and nursing care, with their own specific equipment, specialized human resources and access to other technologies for diagnosis and therapy.

- Intra- and inter-institutional neonatal transport:

Transport of the newborn at risk takes place in the intra-hospital environment, more precisely between the delivery room and the neonatal intermediate or intensive care unit, as well as the neonatal unit and the diagnostic and/or surgical center. Inter-institutional transport usually takes place from a less specialized institution to a more specialized one, after the patient has been stabilized in the hospital of origin, discussed in agreement with the team at the destination hospital, with the vacancy secured. The aim is to improve the patient's survival and quality of life.

- Outpatient clinic for low-risk newborns:

The team must be trained in breastfeeding, and the following are needed to provide care for 8 hours a day: pediatrician with PTE, nurse, nursing assistant, secretary.

- Comprehensive care for the development of newborns at risk:

It consists of an outpatient clinic for newborns weighing less than 1,5000 g, with gestational ages of less than 34 weeks, small for gestational age, suffering from perinatal asphyxia, neurological diseases, congenital infections, among others (RODRIGUES, 2011).

2.9 Humanization

Humanization: act or effect of humanizing. Humanize: make human; give a human condition to, humanize. Humanizing is not a technique, an art and even less an artifice; it is an experiential process that permeates the entire activity of the place and the people who work there, giving the patient the treatment they deserve as a human person, within the peculiar circumstances in which each one finds themselves at the time of their hospitalization. (*AMIB, 2004)*

With the advance of modernity, and technology at its peak, people end up being fascinated by science and techniques, to the point of objectifying people and deifying technology. In order to alleviate this situation, it was necessary to rediscover that we are people and that we don't live alone and that we need each other in order to rediscover humanization.

So the question arises: what is humanization? To humanize is to guarantee dignity and ethics. In order to understand the suffering of others, it is necessary to understand and comprehend dialogue, so humanizing depends on the ability to speak and listen. In other words, without communication there is no humanization.

The growth of technological and scientific development has undoubtedly brought many benefits to society, but it has the adverse effect of increasing dehumanization. A hospital can be the most technologically developed and still be inhumane in its care. This happens when it treats the patient as an object of technical intervention without listening to their anxieties and fears, and often these patients are not even informed of what is being done to them (AMIB, 2004).

The process of massification of industrial society, with an exaggerated valorization of science and technology to the detriment of man and his values, occurred in an unconscious and unreasonable manner in various sectors of society, including the health sector (AMIB, 2004).

Humanization is about individualizing care according to each person's needs. It is important to understand that humanization is not just about changing the physical structure of a hospital, but mainly about changing behaviour and attitudes towards patients and their families. It is true that changing the physical environment is important, but it is not the main focus. Lack of financial resources is not an excuse for not having a humanization programme, but rather the professionals who directly and indirectly assist these patients. In the hospital area, especially the ICU, this process has become more evident because it is the area that concentrates the most technology. Hence the need to integrate humanization with the aim of valuing human characteristics. The starting point was a team aware of the challenges to be faced and the limits to be overcome (AMIB, 2004).

2.11 Humanizing Care

The humanization of health care needs the essence of being, respecting people's individuality and needs. It is therefore understood that the process of humanized care is to make it easier for people who are vulnerable to face their challenges positively. Humanized care aims for the caregiver to understand the meaning of life, giving them the ability to perceive and understand themselves and others. It requires health professionals to share experiences that can be reflected in their actions. Humanizing care is nothing more than giving quality to the professional-patient relationship. It is recognizing and welcoming the anguish of the fragility of the human being in body, mind and spirit (PESSINI; BERTACHINI, 2004).

2.11.1 Ethics and Hospital Humanization

Hospital humanization is generated by many considerations: therapeutic, financial, religious, humanitarian and ethical. It is believed that a person recovers much better from their illness in a pleasant environment where they feel valued as a human being (AMIB, 2004).

> From this perspective, it is important to point out that ethics is not so much concerned with things as they are, but with things as they could be and, above all, as they should be. Ethics dreams of a different world and tries to unravel the logic of the mechanisms that make this dream come true (AMIB, 2004).

Hospitals are often inhumane and end up becoming places where people feel diminished and devalued. In fact, because they are concerned with technical perfection, they end up transforming the patient into a mere object of care, so that the comfort and physical and mental well-being of the sick person end up becoming subordinate to the demands of machines or economic restrictions imposed by the hospital administration. In order to emphasize humanization, the rights and duties of a patient must be imposed within the framework of ethics, such as: the right to medical care; the right to personalized, respectful and caring nursing care; the patient's right to know about the reality of their situation; the patient's right to decide about their life and treatment; and, finally, people's right to a human environment conducive to living and dying with dignity (PESSINI; BERTACHINI, 2004).

2.11.2 Public Policies for Humanization in Health in Brazil

According to Pessini and Bertachini (2004), in Brazil there are programs aimed at humanizing health, one of which is the National Program for the Humanization of Health Services (PNHSS), launched on May 24, 2000, which aims to reduce the difficulties encountered in treatment, favoring the recovery of communication between health professionals and their clients, including the family.

According to the Ministry of Health (2013), in the Unified Health System (SUS), scientific progress, the use of diagnostic devices, surgical techniques and the development of preventive actions have not been accompanied by humanized care. For this reason, the Ministry of Health is proposing a new program aimed at improving personal contact between patients and professionals so that they can be cared for in a more humane and supportive way.

Initially, this project covered eleven hospitals in the public network and included the following phrases: raising awareness, setting up a humanization committee, drawing up action programmes, implementation, evaluation and replanning, respecting the reality of each unit.

Another project is the Prenatal and Birth Humanization Program (Ordinance 569/GM, June 1, 2000), the aim of which is to provide better care in the prenatal, childbirth and puerperium programs. Among its guidelines, it also states that the federal, state and municipal health authorities are responsible for the rights of pregnant women and newborns, in a humanized and safe way.

Another initiative in the field of public policies is the proposal for Humanization in the Family Health Program, implemented by the Ministry of Health in 1994, focusing on humanization under a comprehensive action aimed at the individual and the family, followed by multidisciplinary actions in the health unit, at home and in the community itself (PESSINI; BERTACHINI, 2004).

2.11.3 Humanizing Healthcare

We are currently going through a profound crisis of humanism. On a global scale, we have witnessed advances in politics, technological development, the rights and duties of citizens, family functions, the health and survival of many peoples, among other things.

For there to be humanization in health, it must be necessary to put humanization into practice in society as a whole. Knowing that a violent society interferes in the context of health institutions (PESSINI; BERTACHINI. 2004).

2.11.4 Humanization and intensive care

For humanization to happen, all team members need to be involved. And this process goes beyond technological and pharmacological interventions focused on the patient. It includes assessing the needs of family members, their level of satisfaction with the care provided and preserving the integrity of the patient as a human being.

With the admission of a loved one to an Intensive Care Unit, family members end up depressed and emotionally shaken. Because of this fragility, the patient must be considered unique, having specific needs, values and beliefs. Maintaining and preserving dignity means respecting the principles of morality and the code of ethics.

2.11.4.1 Patient

Patients in an ICU are often dependent and feel a lack of autonomy and self-control. Even though they are surrounded by people, they often still feel anxious and isolated. And when hospital staff ignore the presence of this patient, it increases the degree of anxiety. In order to reduce this feeling, it is important to talk about the treatment through reassuring contact at a time of fear.

Humanizing the ICU means caring for the patient as a whole, encompassing family and society. This practice must bring together everyone's values, hopes, cultural aspects and concerns. In the face of hospitalization, the patient is in a state of fragility and with it comes emotional imbalance.

Patients in the ICU need to be respected and cared for, as (PESSINI; BERTACHIN, 2004).

- Pain control, privacy, individuality, the right to information, to be heard about your complaints and anxieties, a suitable sleeping environment, attention to your modesty, attention to your beliefs and spirituality, the presence of your family, the right to palliative care, the right to compassion.

2.11.4.2 Family

Family is understood to be the social unit that lives in connection with the patient through love and compassion, whether or not there are blood ties. The family is vitally important for the patient's recovery.

The family is a nucleus that needs to be understood as a unit, a system that has internal laws of functioning and organization. And when a family member becomes ill or is hospitalized, it ends up shaking the structures of everyone in the family.

It is necessary for the family to be informed about the onset of the disease, right through to the diagnosis and prognosis, so that they can feel supported, safe and with any doubts clarified. It is important to interview parents or carers during hospitalization in order to obtain information about the patient.

On these occasions, they would provide details about their role and function, reassure the family members, discuss their doubts, establishing a bond between the team and the family. In this way, the team would work together, if possible making the information more consistent, avoiding incomplete conversations and doubts. In these situations, notions of food, diet, hygiene, prognosis, interventions, mental health, contributions from the mother-participant (in the pediatric home) could be presented (AMIB, 2004).

The family needs to talk about the illness, the fears that afflict them, such as death, expressing their feelings to the professional. And when it comes to the ICU, they feel even more helpless because it is an environment in which the patient is subjected to invasive and non-invasive procedures such as tubes, dressings, wires and connected devices, so they feel afraid to touch their loved one for fear of damaging the device and the patient. It is at this point that the team has the opportunity to offer support to the family and the patient, explaining and describing the equipment and the situation in which their loved one is, preparing them to face reality before they get to bed. And touch can be a way of giving the family confidence and support.

2.11.4.3 Team

In order to put humanization into practice, it is essential to understand the team in an interdisciplinary way, acting, empowering and respecting each one.

ICU professionals are confronted with death on a daily basis, which can be related to the cause of occupational stress.

Intercurrences such as changes in the patient's condition increase tension and anxiety, causing concern among the team as a whole. This can lead to frustration, anger, depression and a lack of self-confidence, reducing satisfaction with their work. It is important that the team is attentive and collaborates in interactive work, facilitating the communication process. In order to achieve cohesion among the team, groups can hold scientific meetings, discuss clinical cases, and always seek the best way to care for the patient.

It is important to emphasize that emotional care is the responsibility of the whole team and that the team itself needs to be in an emotional state to work with patients, their families and communities. Small attitudes on the part of professionals can indicate the process of humanization and rescue the dignity of the human being, such as (GUANAES; SOUZA, 2004).

- Call the patient by name, use a calm tone of voice at a normal volume, look at the patient's face and establish courteous and respectful contact, address the patient whenever you approach the bed for a procedure, examine the patient in an attentive manner, use gentle touch.

2.11.5 . Humanization in the Pediatric ICU

Pediatric Intensive Care Units (PICUs) emerged in the 1960s, with ever-increasing technological development and the possibility of better conditions for rapid diagnosis, continuous monitoring and early and efficient curative interventions. This led to the emergence of increasingly specialized professionals who were able to master this technology, and the need to create new protocols and strict routines in order to speed up data collection and procedures in order to cure diseases.

It's true that the infant mortality rate has dropped considerably, but the emphasis on the dominance of illness and death has perhaps erased the recognition that the PICU is an environment of isolation and anxiety, depersonalization, stress and hyperstimulation for both patients and professionals (AMIB, 2004).

The patient becomes a number on a bed or in a medical record, a syndrome or a diseased organ, rather than a human being with psycho-emotional needs who is suffering because of the illness and because of being cut off from their environment and family (AMIB, 2004).

The multidisciplinary team becomes responsible for efficiency, for not making mistakes, being there at all times in an attempt to intervene in death with the aim of saving lives. The family suffers because of the separation, the illness of their loved one and what might happen due to the lack of information. However, this has led medical and nursing professionals to realize that there should be changes in the care of sick children, their families and the multidisciplinary team, calling it the humanization of ICUs.

The major trigger for humanization was the Declaration of the Rights of Hospitalized Children and Adolescents (Resolution No. 41 of the Ministry of Justice and the National Council for the Rights of Children and Adolescents, October 1995). (AMIB, 2004)

Humanizing is not as difficult or as rare as it may seem. All that is needed is for each professional to carry out their role with sensitivity, goodwill, creativity and efficiency, seeking the recovery, preservation and satisfaction of the child, the family and the team, with a view to respecting and maintaining the integrity of the human being (AMIB, 2004).

2.11.6 Humanization in the Neonatal ICU

It is known that newborns, regardless of their gestational age at birth, are capable of expressing pain and pleasure, as well as seeking "contact" or fleeing from it when stress is generated (PEREIRA. Pg. 33, 2011).

Care in the neonatal ICU should be aimed at providing the neonate with well-being, as well as reducing the degree of stress for the baby themselves and their families. Some measures should be taken to improve this, with a view to the humanized aspect, such as:

A) Freeing up visiting hours for parents: extending visiting hours for parents favors the newborn's emotional ties and future social relationships.

B) Adoption of "parent information hours": in addition to improving the work routine of professionals, as it prevents parents from being interrupted repeatedly to find out information about their children, it also makes parents feel more secure in their relationship with the health professional. They will know the right time to receive information about their children and will be able to ask any questions they may have. In addition, they will receive information whenever possible from the same doctor, the one who takes care of the newborn on a daily basis, creating a better relationship between doctor and family.

C) Visiting hours for grandparents: allows other family members, in this case the grandparents, to accompany the treatment of the newborn, improving the emotional relationship between them.

D) Identifying the newborn by name: the fact that parents have to deal with the disappointment of not having had a healthy newborn like the one they dreamed of can cause a certain degree of rejection of the sick newborn. This procedure brings parents closer to the baby they idealized during pregnancy, promoting greater acceptance of the real baby.

E) Identifying parents by name: the simple fact of calling parents by name creates an individualization of the person and their child, leading to a sense of respect and consideration for the family on the part of health professionals.

F) Weekly meetings with parents ("parents' group"): these meetings discuss general topics in the unit, as well as clearing up any doubts about the sector's progress. Parents also have the opportunity to talk to each other, exchanging experiences from their day-to-day life in the school.

G) Snooze time: you should establish times when newborns are left without any kind of manipulation, with lighting reduced as much as possible and noise reduced as much as possible.

H) Implementation of the Kangaroo Mother method (humanized care for preterm newborns): this is a set of measures adopted by the Ministry of Health with the aim of promoting the humanization of perinatal care, as well as encouraging breastfeeding. The implementation of these measures and others that contribute to the well-being of the newborn makes perinatal care safe, of quality and at the same time supportive and humanized (PEREIRA, 2011).

2.11.6.1 How the Standard of Humanized Care for Low Birth Weight Newborns (Kangaroo Method/Ministry of Health) came about

In July 1999, almost a year after research and observation, the Ministry of Health drew up a draft with the aim of humanizing care for low birth weight babies. This project brought together representatives from various organizations such as: Brazilian Society of Pediatrics, Brazilian Federation of Gynecology and Obstetrics, Pan American Health Organization (PAHO), United Nations Children's Fund (UNICEF), as well as representatives from Brazilian universities (University of Brasilia (UnB) and Federal University of Rio de Janeiro (UFRJ), the Maternal and Child Institute of Pernambuco (IMIP), the State Health Secretariats of the Federal District and the States of São Paulo and technicians from the

Women's Health Area of the SPS/MS. This led to the creation of the HUMANIZED ATTENTION TO THE LOW WEIGHT NEWBORN (CANGURU METHOD). On December 8, 1999, it was officially presented by the Minister of State for Health, José Serra (OLIVEIRA, 2006).

On March 2, 2000, the Ministry of Health published ordinance number 72: "Norma de Orientaçâo para Implantaçâo do Projeto Kanguru", regulating remuneration for this type of care in the Hospital Admissions System of the Unified Health System (SIH/SUS). (OLIVEIRA, 2006)

2.11.6.2 What is the Ministry of Health's Humanized Care Standard?

Unlike the idealized model of the Colony in the late 1970s, the Kangaroo Method aims to change the way the mother, family and professionals involved care for the low-birth-weight newborn, with the aim of humanizing care. Skin-to-skin contact is established at an early stage between mother and low-birth-weight newborn in an incremental manner and for as long as they both feel is pleasurable and sufficient, thus allowing parents to participate more in the newborn's care (OLIVEIRA, 2006).

This gradual contact can evolve into placing the child in the kangaroo position, which is where the baby lies prone, in an upright position, against the chest of an adult, who may be the mother, father or possibly another family member. Adopting these measures encourages greater attachment, security, breastfeeding and better development of the child (OLIVEIRA, 2006).

The standard does not advocate replacing modern technologies in the care of newborns at risk, but instead establishes important and current concepts, constituting a new and modern vision of care. The Brazilian method is designed to be developed in three stages, one interconnected to the other, so that the next stage is based on the adequate work of the previous stage.

2.11.6.2.1 First stage

It starts with identifying pregnant women at risk of giving birth to a low birth weight child. Once this situation has been confirmed, the mother-to-be receives specific guidance on how to care for herself and her baby. As soon as the baby is born and needs to be kept in a neonatal intensive care unit and/or intermediate care, special attention is needed to encourage the parents to enter the unit. From there, we work on lactation and the participation of family members together, establishing skin-to-skin contact. The kangaroo position should be offered whenever possible.

2.11.6.2.2 Second stage

In the second stage, the baby is in a stable clinical situation, has gained weight regularly for at least three days and weighs more than 1,250g. The mother is safe, there is family and institutional support and it is in the mother's interest to remain in the rooming-in unit where the kangaroo position can be practiced for as long as both find it pleasant. The vigilance of the health team is fundamental to the success of the project.

2.11.6.2.3 Third stage

The third stage takes place outside the hospital, with outpatient follow-up, and only occurs if the child weighs at least 1,500 g at the time of discharge, is clinically stable, and is gaining weight while breastfeeding. It is important that the mother and family members keep their newborn at home in the kangaroo position 24 hours a day. Generally, at around 2,500 g, the kangaroo position is no longer used (OLIVEIRA, 2006).

3 METHODOLOGY

3.1 TYPE OF STUDY AND RESEARCH METHOD

A qualitative, descriptive field study will be carried out to observe and record the daily lives of nurses on duty in the neonatal intensive care unit, with the aim of understanding the meaning of humanization for each of the professionals studied, based on Bardin's method.

3.2 LOCATION/CONNECTION

It was founded in the 1650s. Its foundation is a direct administration body, linked to the State Secretariat for Public Health and certified as a teaching hospital. Currently the new building has been inaugurated, with 406 new beds installed in an area of 22,000 square meters, the complex has 8 floors, with beds distributed in the pediatrics, neonatology and maternal ICU wards.

and pediatric ward, maternity ward, intermediate care unit (ICU), ward for the "Kangaroo Mother" program and obstetric reception.

It is the oldest health institution in the north of Brazil, and its essential purposes are: Care, Teaching and Research, in line with the Care Profile in Child Health Care, Women's Health Care, Adult Health Care, providing outpatient and inpatient services. It is a hospital that provides 100% SUS services and is registered as a reference for high-risk pregnant women and newborns.

In the area of teaching and research, it runs medical residency programs in Pediatrics, Neonatology, Pediatric Nephrology, Gynecology and Obstetrics, Internal Medicine, Dermatology, General Surgery, Pediatric Surgery and Radiology. Its mission is to provide quality, humanized health care for women and children, acting as a general hospital and as a teaching and research hospital, in conjunction with public policies.

3.3 CRITERIA FOR INCLUSION IN THE STUDY

Nurses working in the neonatal intensive care unit on duty in the morning, afternoon and evening shifts will be included in the study.

3.4 RESEARCH SUBJECT EXCLUSION CRITERIA

Nurses from the morning, afternoon and night shifts who are on medical leave, those who are not on duty on the day of the survey and nurses from other sectors will be excluded from the survey.

3.5 DATA COLLECTION TECHNIQUE(S)

Data will be collected through semi-structured interviews containing open-ended questions. The answers will be collected using a tape recorder.

3.6 DATA ANALYSIS TECHNIQUE(S)

We will use Bardin's (1977) Content Analysis, which is characterized by a set of methodological tools that are applied to extremely diverse discourses (contents and continents), in which we will use the qualitative model.

3.7 ETHICAL ASPECTS

It was sent to the Ethics Committee, introducing the researchers and requesting authorization to carry out the research in the Neonatal Intensive Care Unit, as well as formalizing the aspects of reliability and confidentiality and the commitment to inform the service of the results of the research. The entire cost of the research will be borne by the researchers, without sponsorship or assistance of any kind from individuals and/or companies.

4 REFERENCES

BRAZILIAN ASSOCIATION OF INTENSIVE CARE MEDICINE. *Humanizaçâo em Cuidados Intensivos/* Livraria e Editora Revinter Ltda, 2004.

BAPTISTA, Tatiana. *Humanization, Gender, Power:* Contributions of Speech Studies in Interaction to Health Care. Rio de Janeiro, 2012.

BERELSON, B. *Content analysis in communication research*. New York: Hafner; 1984

BERTACHINI, Luciana. PESSINI, Leo. *Humanization and Palliative Care* - 5 Ed. - Loyola Jesuitas, Sâo Paulo, 2004.

BRAZIL. Ministry of Health. *HumanizaSUS:* national humanization policy. Brasilia, 2013.

FONTES, Paulo. *Ethics, users' rights and policies for humanizing health care. 2004.*

OLIVEIRA, Beatriz. LOPES, Thais. VIERA, Clàudia. COLLET, Neusa. *The work process of the neonatal ICU nursing team and care*

humanized.2006

OLIVEIRA, Isabel. RODRIGUES, Renata. *Newborn Care:* Perspectives for Nursing Knowledge in Neonatology (1937-1979), 2005.

PEREIRA, Caroline. MIRANDA, Livia. PASSOS, Joanir. *The occupational stress of nursing in a closed sector. 2009.*

PINTO, T. M. Filosofia em enfermagem:algumas reflexôes. Pelotas: UFPel; 1998.

POTTER, Patricia. PERRY, Anne. Fundamentals of Nursing. Rio de Janeiro. 2012.

RODRIGUES, F. P; MAGALHAES, M. *Normas e condutas em neonatologia /* editors. -2.ed. - Sao Paulo: Editora Atheus, 2011.

SA, Lopes. *Professional Ethics - 6.ed.- Sâo Paulo: Atlas, 2005.*

SALICIO, Dalvia. GAVIA, Maria. *The meaning of humanizing care for ICU nurses.* 2006

SOUZA, Kâtia. FERREIRA, Suely. *Humanized care in the neonatal ICU:* the meanings and limitations identified by health professionals. Rio de Janeiro, 2008.

SOUZA, Maria. SARTOR, Vicente. PRADO, Marta. *Subsidies for an Ethic of Responsibility in Nursing,* 2005.

TOMEZ, R. SILVA, M. *Nursing in the Neonatal ICU. 1.ed. Rio de Janeiro. 2006.*

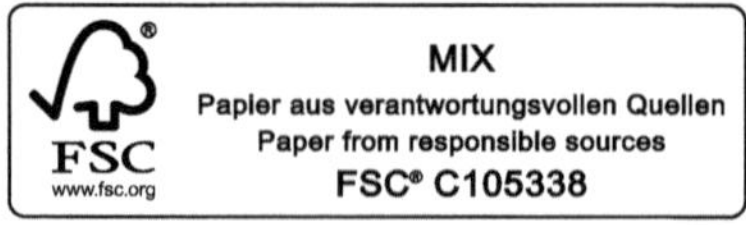

Printed by Books on Demand GmbH, Norderstedt / Germany